PILATES
for men

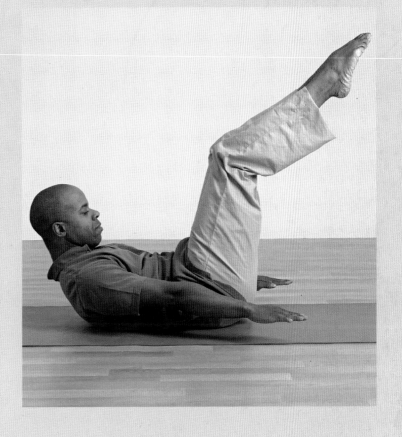

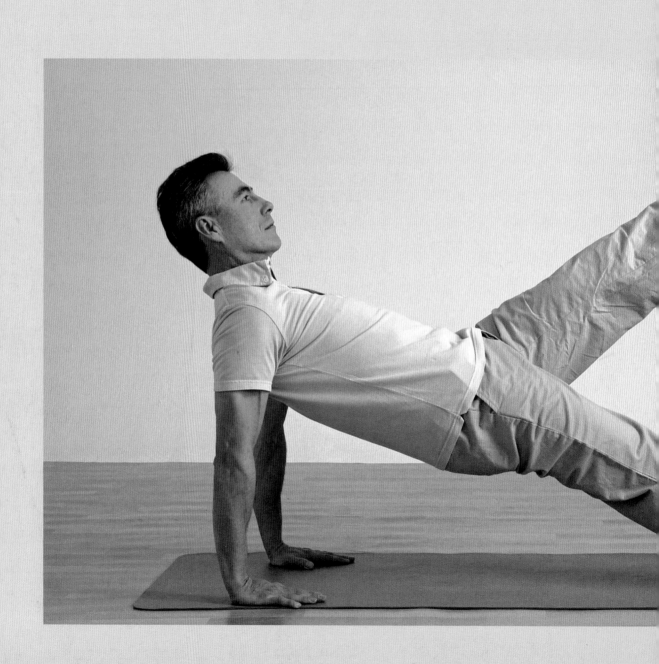

PILATES
for men

fit for sport
fit for life

ALAN HERDMAN
with Gill Paul

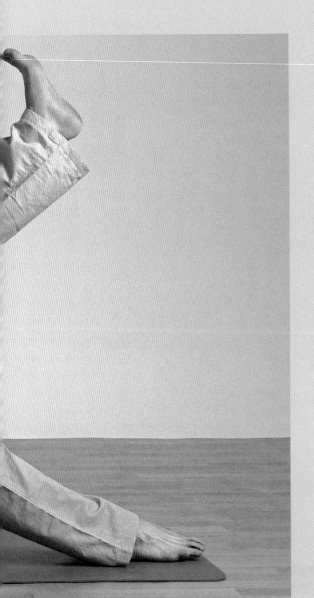

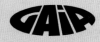

Reconnect with yourself and the planet

First published in Great Britain in 2007 by Gaia Books
a division of Octopus Publishing Group Ltd
2–4 Heron Quays, London, E14 4JP.

Distributed in the United States and Canada by
Sterling Publishing Co., Inc.
387 Park Avenue South, New York, NY 10016–8810

ISBN-13: 978-185675-268-8
ISBN-10: 1-85675-268-2

A CIP catalogue record of this book is available from
the British Library.

Printed and bound in China

10 9 8 7 6 5 4 3 2 1

Caution

This book is not intended to replace medical care under the
direct supervision of a qualified doctor. Before embarking on
any changes in your health regime, consult your doctor. While
all the techniques, ideas and suggestions detailed in this book
are extremely safe if done correctly, you must seek professional
advice if you are in any doubt about any medical condition.

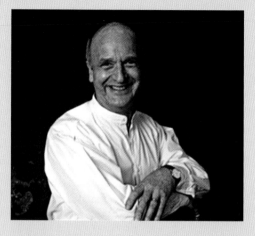

About the author

I learned the Pilates method from two of
Joseph Pilates' protégés, Bob Fitzgerald and
Carola Trier, just after Joseph Pilates died in
1967, and I brought it across the Atlantic to
open the UK's first Pilates studio in 1970.
Since then, I have continued to adapt and
develop new exercises to address the needs of
every client I consult with. I have worked with
actors, dancers, musicians, doctors, dentists,
journalists, builders and sportsmen and
women – all kinds of people with a huge
variety of physical problems. I use a piece of
equipment called a 'reformer' in my studio
– a kind of supportive exercise machine with
springs, based on the prototypes Pilates
developed – but I always train each client in
mat work first. This means that they have an
understanding of all the correct techniques
required to be able to do Pilates at home.
Sometimes new problems call for new
solutions, but the principles that Joseph Pilates
established in the early 20th century remain
the core of my work.

Contents

Introduction

The exercise system that Joseph Pilates invented back in the early 20th century was used to help soldiers to rehabilitate from wounds sustained in World War 1, and then became the method of choice for dancers trying to remain supple to avoid injury. It subsequently gained popularity with actors, TV performers, injury-prone athletes and those who found their desk jobs were playing havoc with their backs. Now, in the 21st century, it is the single most effective system for smoothing out the aches and pains caused by the fast pace of modern life, and its popularity increases all the time.

Joseph Pilates initially designed the exercises for himself. His body was twisted and stunted from childhood rickets, rheumatic fever and asthma, but with a mixture of intuition, dedication and sheer hard work, he transformed himself into a professional boxer, circus performer, self-defence instructor, gymnast and all-round health guru. This may sound incredible, but anyone who tries Pilates exercises for even a few sessions will see changes for the better. Muscles grow more defined, posture improves, stomachs become flatter, joints are looser and more flexible – and the harder you work, the better it gets.

I still use many of the original exercises Pilates taught. The Intermediate and Advanced routines described in this book contain many examples from his famous repertoire, known as 'The 34'. I learned the system from two of his disciples in New York in the late 1960s, and when I came back to the UK I was the first to introduce Pilates to these shores. Over the decades I've added some new exercises and adapted original ones to deal with the wide range of problems clients consult me about in my studio – and believe me, I've seen some strange cases in my time.

Pilates doesn't involve pumping iron, performing dozens of mindless repetitions, or even breaking a sweat. You do, however, need to concentrate hard to coordinate your movements and breathing, line yourself up precisely so that exactly the right muscle group is used, and create 'muscle memories' so that you know what to do to achieve optimum results next time. Pilates exercises are performed slowly and rhythmically. You start on the simplest moves and only progress when you can complete them impeccably. Leave your competitive instincts at work or on the football pitch!

Who is Pilates good for? Anyone who gets back pain or joint problems; those who use their bodies for their work, such as actors, dancers and sportsmen; people who haven't exercised for years and dread exposing flabby muscles in a gym; and anyone who wants their body to look the very best it can possibly be. If this sounds like you, read on.

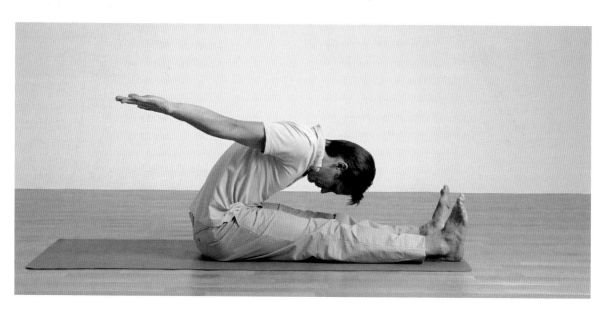

The basic principles of Pilates

The principles I teach in my studio today were developed from the original ones Joseph Pilates taught, but I've dropped a few of his more extreme instructions (such as exercising outdoors in midwinter wearing only a pair of bathing trunks). Still, I think you'll find the system quite different from any other form of exercise you've ever tried. Here are the basic rules:

Concentration

Forget about work, money, sex or whatever else is on your mind. You can't do Pilates effectively without focusing exclusively on the way your body is feeling and how your muscles respond to the movements.

Control

It's better to complete one perfect Pilates movement than ten sloppy ones. Flicking through this book, you may think some exercises look easy, but you'll find that it can take weeks of practice to perform even the simplest ones accurately, with complete control of all the muscle groups.

Centre

Many Pilates exercises focus on strengthening the muscles of the abdomen, hips and buttocks, because a strong centre is the key to protecting the spine and stabilizing the rest of the body.

Fluidity

Movements should be smooth and flowing, with no straining, jerking, heaving, panting or grunting. During your exercise routine each exercise should be performed with a sense of purpose.

Precision

In a Pilates studio, instructors will correct your position as you work because if you are only a couple of centimetres out of alignment the movement will be much less effective. If you are teaching yourself with the help of this book, you will have to check and recheck your position before and during each exercise, or get a critical friend to help. Less is usually better than more, so aim for small, clean movements rather than large imprecise ones.

Breathing

During Pilates exercises you breathe in through your nose and out through your mouth. In general, you breathe out on the effort part of the exercise, or as you move away from the centre of the body, and breathe in during preparation or on the return to the centre, but check the specific breathing instructions with each exercise. They make an important contribution to the effectiveness of the movements.

Imagination

If you can visualize a movement in your mind's eye, it is easier to isolate the muscles that will achieve it. Just thinking about your abdominal muscles controlling a movement will often help you to activate them.

Intuition

As you learn Pilates, you will learn more about your body – its strengths, weaknesses, asymmetries and capabilities. So, when a movement feels difficult or you get a twinge in a joint, you will understand how to self-diagnose and take action to fix it yourself. Awareness of your body will also help you to judge when a problem requires medical advice.

Integration

There are many different things to think about during even the simplest Pilates exercise. You need to be aware of the position of every part of your body, including the bits that you're not working; you need to think about breathing correctly, activating the muscles required for the movement, then performing the sequence of actions and counting the number of repetitions. You must make sure that you are only working the muscles that are supposed to be working, and can't feel strain anywhere else. To do all this, work slowly and rhythmically.

Chapter 1
Assess yourself

Pilates is not just about doing some exercise two or three times a week. The real benefits come when you extend the theory into everyday life and learn to use correct posture at home, at work, in the car and playing sport. This chapter is about assessing what your body is like now and identifying any bad habits you may have developed over the years (postural, that is – I don't want to know about the others).

Twelve tests of strength and flexibility

How fit are you? I'm not asking if you would be able to run a marathon tomorrow or take part in a squash tournament next weekend. In Pilates, the aim is to be fit for everyday life so that your muscles are strong enough to control your joints correctly as you undertake normal day-to-day activities. You should be able to lift a packed box without straining your lower back, put your socks and trousers on in the morning without sitting on the edge of the bed and dig up a flowerbed without having to lie on a sofa moaning afterwards. Now do you think you are fit?

Try the following tests, then add up your score to see how fit you are in Pilates' terms. Take note of any movements you can't manage because the next chapter will analyze problem areas and suggest solutions.

1 Sit on the floor with your legs out straight in front of you, shoulder-width apart, and with your spine straight. Rest your hands on your knees. Now bend forwards from the waist and award yourself two points if you can touch your ankle bones. If you can actually hold onto the soles of your feet while keeping your legs straight, you get four points, but bend from the waist and don't curve your upper back forwards.

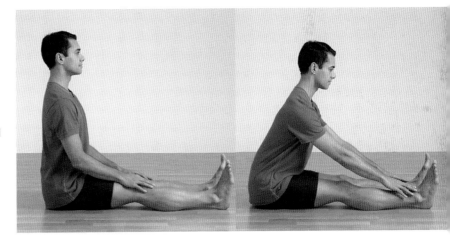

2 Stand facing a mirror with your feet one hip-width apart. With your arms out to your sides to help you balance, raise one leg for 30 seconds; now stand on the other leg for 30 seconds. Try this with your eyes closed. One tip: don't lean into one hip or you'll lose your balance – try to keep your hips level. Take two points if you can stand on both your left and your right leg with your eyes open; and an extra five points if you can do it with your eyes closed.

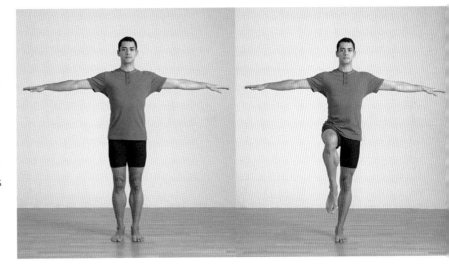

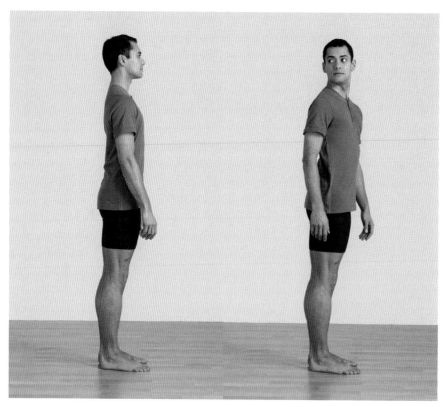

3 Stand with your back to a mirror. Keeping your hips still, turn your upper body to the right. Can you see into the mirror behind you without moving your hips? Now turn your upper body to the left. Award yourself two points if you can see into the mirror from both the left and the right.

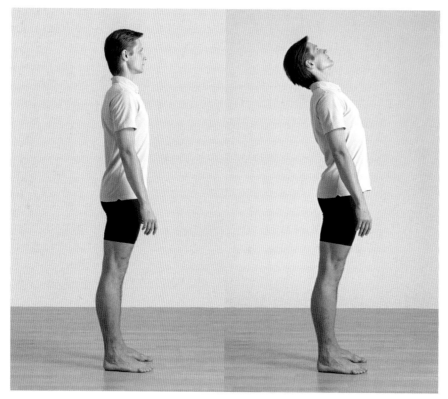

4 Standing up straight look up at the ceiling and think about where you are curving your spine to do so. Is it your waist, upper back or neck, or all three? Take one point for each part of your spine that is mobile.

5 Stand facing the mirror. Take a deep breath in and watch where your breath goes, and make sure you don't raise your shoulders when you breathe (see far right). Deduct two points from your score if your shoulders rise at all.

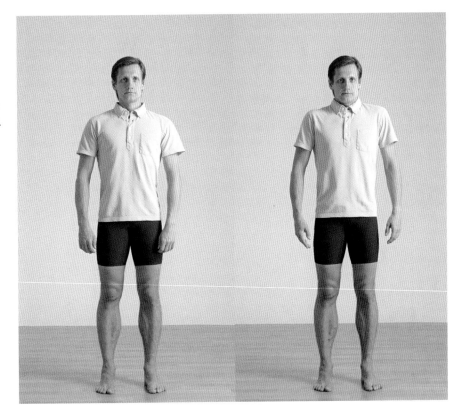

6 Stand straight in front of the mirror with your arms by your sides. Breathe in, pull in your stomach muscles and bend over to your left, keeping your hips facing squarely forwards. Can you bend far enough so that your fingers are level with your knee? Now try bending to your right. Take four points if your fingertips reach your knees on both sides.

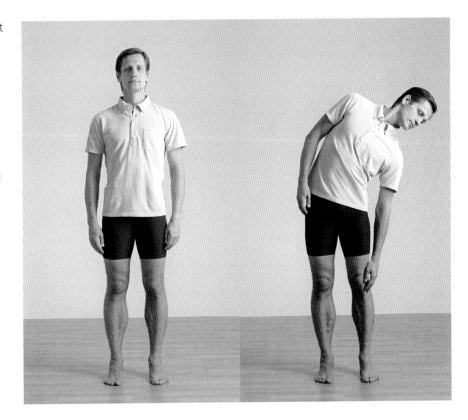

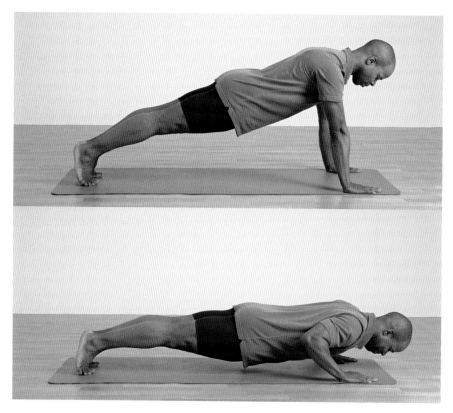

7 Lie on the floor and raise up on your toes and hands, arms straight. Can you do a press-up, keeping your spine in a straight line? Bend your elbows to lower your body to within 5 cm (2 in) of the floor, keeping your elbows by your sides, then push back up again. You get three points for a successful press-up.

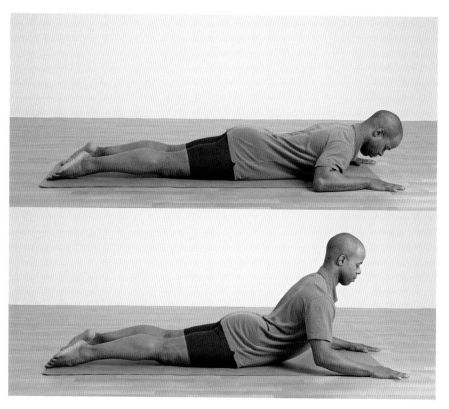

8 Lie face down with your palms on the floor at chest level and your elbows pointing outwards. Lift your upper body from the floor so that it forms a C-shaped curve and hold for ten seconds. Is every part of your spine curving – the lower (lumbar), upper (thoracic) and neck (cervical)? Some people have a tendency to strain back with their neck if the thoracic spine is immobile. Award yourself two points if you are curving your spine in all three areas.

9 Lie face down on the floor again, with your palms at head level and knees together. Bend your right leg and catch hold of your right foot with your right hand. Can you pull it back so that the heel touches your bottom without your hips moving off the floor? Repeat with the right foot. If you can do it on both sides you get two points.

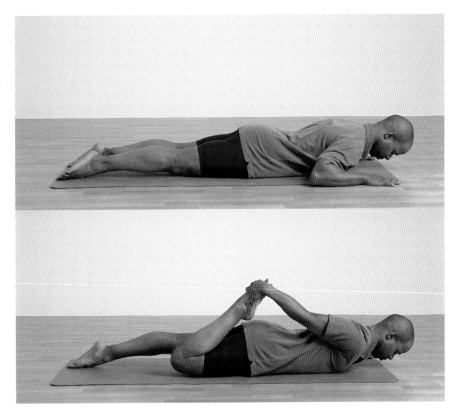

10 Stand up straight with your arms out in front of you at shoulder level, palms facing down. Your hips, knees and ankles should be aligned with each other. Bend your knees in a half squat at an angle of roughly 45 degrees, keeping your spine straight. Don't bend forwards, raise your shoulders or lift your heels off the floor. Take two points if you can do this. Now try a full squat all the way down to the floor. Your heels will rise slightly, but your back should stay straight and the movement should be smooth. If you can do this, take another three points.

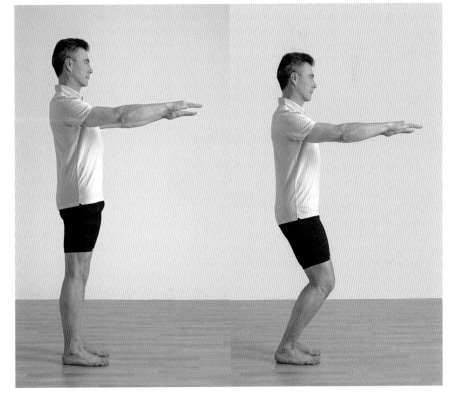

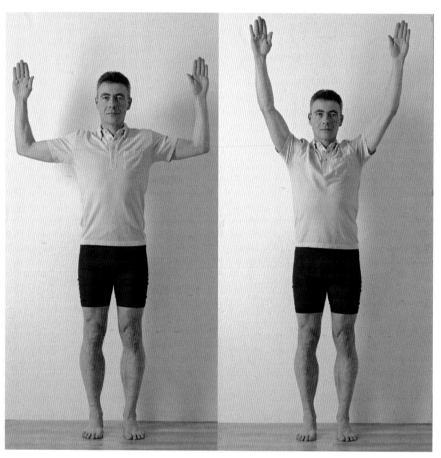

11 Stand with your hips, shoulders and head against a wall and your feet about 15 cm (6 in) away from the wall. Bend your elbows at 90 degrees and rest them against the wall at shoulder level, with your forearms and hands vertical against the wall above. Slide your arms up the wall, keeping your elbows and forearms against it, until your arms are straight. If your head, forearms or elbows lose contact with the wall at any stage, you get no points; if you manage to straighten and maintain contact, take three points.

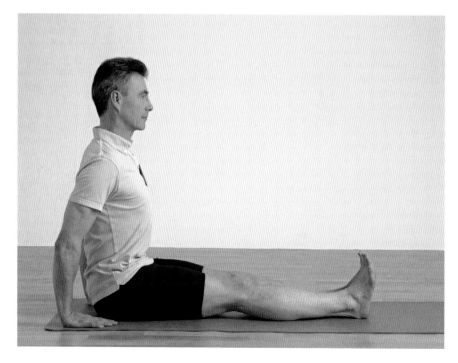

12 Sit up straight and pull your abdominal muscles towards your spine. Are you able to make your stomach flat, or even concave? You get two points for flat; four points for concave.

Adding up your scores

Under 15

You're as stiff as a plank of wood! Either you haven't exercised at all since your school days, or you have been focusing on a sport that builds up one set of muscles instead of providing all-round flexibility. It doesn't sound as though you're the kind of guy who can get his socks on in the morning while standing up – in fact, you may not have been able to touch your toes for some time. I wonder who cuts your toenails for you? You need to start by strengthening your postural muscles, but take it very gently. No leaping ahead to advanced Pilates routines; slowly and carefully are the 'watch' words.

15–30

You probably thought you were quite fit, but there are obviously some areas that need attention. Was it the shoulders, lower back or hamstrings that let you down? Did you find you were asymmetrical, able to manage a movement on one side but not the other? All these clues are important to figure out exactly what is going on with your body and which areas you need to strengthen. Read on, because the posture check on pages 16 and 17 may throw up a few more enlightening facts.

Over 30

Not bad at all. If you got full marks (39 points), you are in pretty good shape. If not, consider the challenge or challenges you couldn't manage and think about which muscles might need to be stretched or strengthened. You probably have good posture already, but continue with the examination in the next section to see where the quirks might be. We all have them!

Check your posture

Another reality check, but this time you have to examine your posture in a full-length mirror. It's best to do this naked or stripped down to your underwear. There's no point in cheating, so I recommend that you get an objective partner or an *extremely* close friend to give a second opinion.

Stand sideways on to the mirror and check the following:
- Does your gut stick out? (Don't pull it in – stand with your normal posture.)
- Does your bottom stick out?
- Look at the shape of your spine. Does the lower back curve inwards? Or does it seem reasonably straight with natural spinal curves, as in the photograph (see below left) showing correct posture?
- Does your chin jut out or tilt upwards?
- Does your upper back curl forwards and are your shoulders hunched?

It should be possible to drop a plumbline from behind your ear, through the shoulder, hip and knee joints, to hit the floor just beside the ankle. Where would your plumbline go? If your pelvis is behind the line, you may have a condition known as kyphosis (see page 24); if it's in front of the line, you may have lordosis (see page 23).

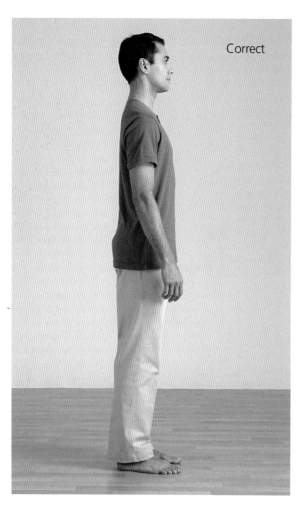

Correct

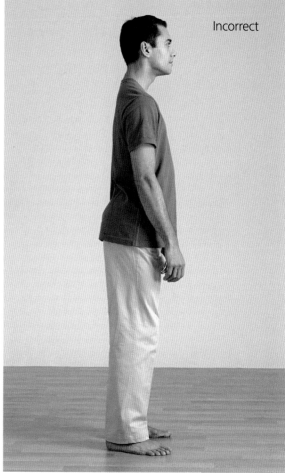

Incorrect

Face the mirror and check the following:
- Is one shoulder higher or one shoulder wider than the other from the neck to the top of the arm?
- As your arms hang by your sides, are the fingers of one hand parallel to the fingers of the other hand?
- Is the gap between your lower arm and hips equal on both sides?
- Are your hip bones level?
- Are your legs straight or bowed? Do your knees touch?

A plumbline running down from your nose and passing through your breastbone and pubic bone should divide you into two symmetrical halves.

One-sided activities

Some professions, such as surgery and dentistry, require you to use one side of your body much more than the other, and those who work on computers can find they develop extra tension in the area of whichever arm they use to hold the mouse. It is the same for sportsmen, golfers and cricketers, for example.

If you can't avoid one-sided activities, make sure you compensate for them during your Pilates workouts by stretching the overworked side and strengthening the muscles of the underused side. Specific advice on this is given in chapter 5 when we look at individual sports.

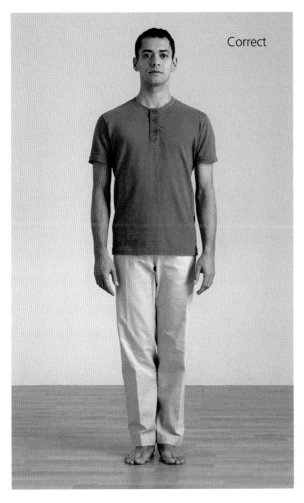

Correct

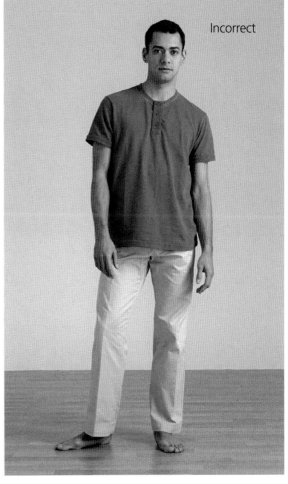

Incorrect

Balance check

Are you balancing your weight evenly through your feet?

Your weight should be distributed in a triangle shape, with the apex at the front of the heel just below the ankle joint, and the base across the pads of your foot before the toe joints. If you are leaning backwards, you might find that you have to lift your toes off the ground for balance. If you lean forwards, your toes will bend like claws to support your weight. Are your toes straight? Some people roll their weight to the insides of their feet, causing knock-kneed postures; others roll to the outsides of their feet, giving bow-legged postures. If you're not sure how you balance your weight, check an old pair of shoes.

• Did they wear out evenly across the soles and heels?
• Or are they more worn under the balls of your feet, under the heels or to the insides or outsides? This could give you a clue as to how your weight is normally distributed while you are standing, walking or running in day-to-day life.

Are you tensing any muscles as you stand straight in front of the mirror?

Do a quick check. Your knees should be straight, but not locked, and about hip-width apart. Both your feet should be firmly on the ground with the weight balanced through the triangle shape. Your stomach should be comfortably held in rather than protruding, your shoulders should be relaxed, and your neck should be long, with your chin parallel to the floor and pulled slightly backwards.

If you feel uncomfortable standing in this position, it means that you need to tone all your muscle groups to hold you up properly. However, there's no point in only adopting the correct posture when you're standing in front of a mirror consciously thinking about it. It needs to become second nature if you are to maintain good posture for life. In the following section, there are descriptions of the correct and incorrect ways of doing some common everyday activities.

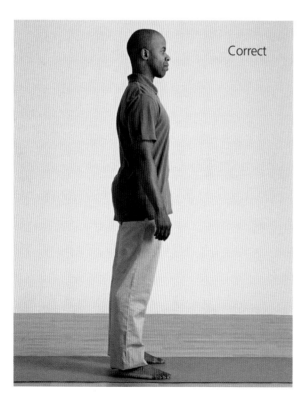

Correct

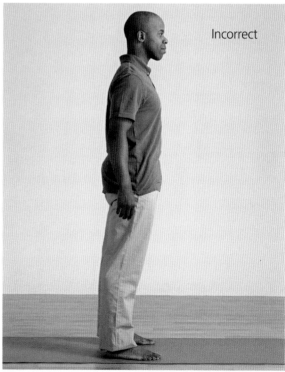

Incorrect

Posture checks in everyday life

Workstation ergonomics

If you have a desk job, look carefully at the way your workstation is set up.

Correct
- You should be able to sit on your chair with your feet on the floor and your knees and hip joints bent at right angles. Your bottom should be positioned right into the back of the chair.
- Your desk should be directly in front of you, and high enough so that you can rest your forearms on it with your elbows bent at right angles and your upper arms at your sides.
- The computer screen should be positioned directly in front of you with the centre of the screen at eye level.
- You should be able to type on your keyboard with your elbows at your sides, and there should be plenty of space to manipulate the mouse and rest your forearm on the desk in between.
- If you spend a lot of time on the telephone, get a hands-free model.
- If you have to do a lot of reading at a desk, get a tilted drawing board.

Incorrect
- Don't cross your legs or sit with your legs twisted round each other.
- Make sure your knees aren't higher than your hips.
- Don't have your feet dangling from a seat that is too high.
- Don't position your computer to one side so that you have to swivel round to work on it.
- Don't hold the telephone between your ear and your shoulder while doing other things as you speak.
- Don't hunch forwards over paperwork.

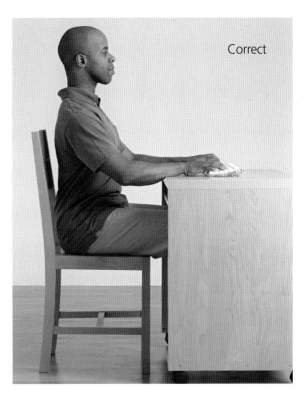

Correct

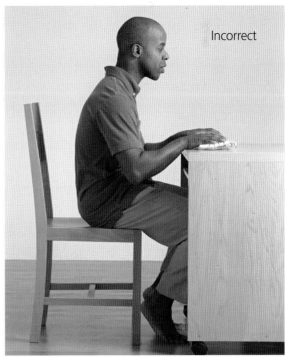

Incorrect

Driving

When you add up the average time that you spend behind the wheel of your car each day it can be significant – bad postural habits will have a cumulative effect on your body.

Correct

- Adjust the car seat so that you can hold the steering wheel with your upper arms at your sides and with your elbows bent at right angles.
- Your knees and hips should also be bent at right angles, the pedals within easy reach, and your back supported by the back of the seat.
- Adjust the rear-view mirror so that you can see into it without stretching, leaning over or turning your head.
- Keep your shoulders relaxed.
- When you are at a stop, put the handbrake on and give your legs a rest.
- On a long drive, stop every two hours to have a walk.
- If you are prone to hip problems, keep your driving to a minimum.

Incorrect

- Don't hunch your shoulders forwards over the wheel in the classic 'road rage' posture.
- Don't rest one arm on the windowsill; keep both hands on the wheel.
- Don't ride the clutch at traffic lights – it's bad for the car and for your legs.
- If you have an automatic car, be careful not to sink your weight into your left hip while your right foot does all the pedal work.
- Your knees shouldn't be higher than your hips.
- Don't twist round to lift briefcases or other items from the back seat – you might put your back out.

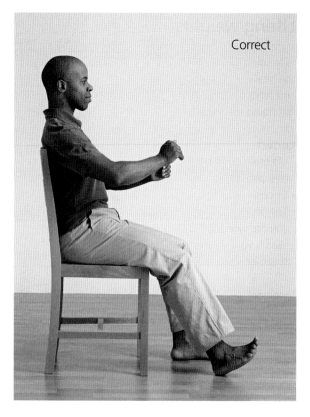

Correct

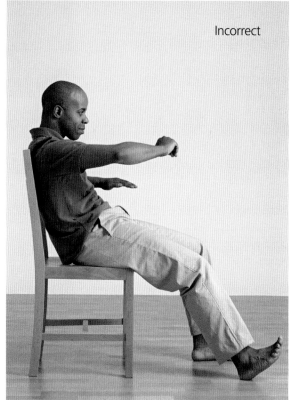

Incorrect

Lifting weights in the gym

I sometimes shudder when I see men in a gym lifting the heaviest weights they can manage while their veins and tendons pop out of their neck and arms. They're not doing themselves any good at all.

Correct
• Maintain good posture with your body weight centred (see also pages 92).
• Choose lighter weights and do more repetitions.
• The only part of the body that should move is the area you are working.
• Watch yourself in a mirror so you can see if there's any strain in your neck.

Incorrect
• Don't use your shoulders to lift.
• When picking up weights, don't lean forwards to reach them and never twist round to pick them up from one side.
• Don't try to lift a weight that causes you to strain.
• Never pick up weights with a rounded back.

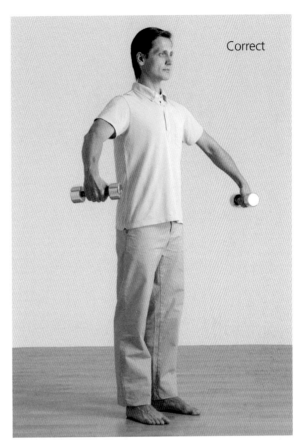

Correct

Throughout the day

Keep monitoring your posture whenever you remember during the day: standing in a queue in the bank, sitting in a traffic jam, watching TV or playing sport. Think of the position of your spine – is it long and tall, with only natural curves, or is it scrunched up in an S shape? Every time you correct your posture by standing tall or sitting up straight, you are strengthening your posture muscles just a little bit. And it's very important to keep them strong if you still want to play sport in your fifties, gardening in your sixties and riding a motorbike across Australia in your seventies (or whatever your retirement ambition might be).

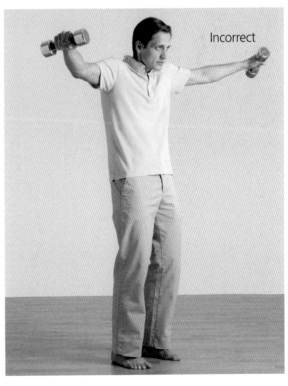

Incorrect

Chapter 2
What can go wrong?

If you thought the last chapter was personal, now we're really getting down to the nitty-gritty. Answer the questions in this chapter and read the sections that apply to you to find out about the physical imbalances you may have developed, and how Pilates can help you to correct them. Keep the results of your Chapter 1 challenges and posture assessment to hand – they may help you to nail down the problems.

Evaluating yourself

This is about being honest with yourself about the aches and pains you usually try to ignore. Feeling stiff after gardening or playing sport doesn't mean the onset of middle age – it just means that you need to strengthen certain muscle groups and look after yourself a bit better.

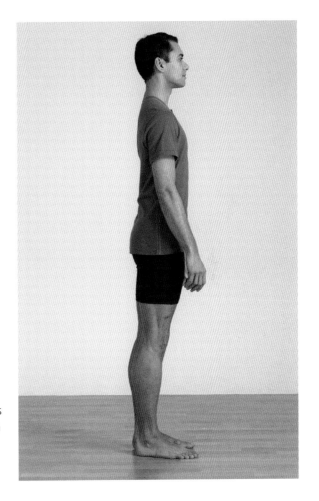

How tall are you?

When did you last get measured? If you haven't checked your height for a few years, measure yourself now (without standing on tiptoes). Are you as tall as you were at the age of 20?

A lot of men are walking around thinking they're six feet tall when they've actually shrunk half an inch or an inch. Unless you've been maintaining perfect posture most of the time, your spine will have been degenerating since your twenties, or even your teens. Studies show that most people in the West have some degree of spinal curvature by the age of 25 – and this is going to make you shorter. It can also lead to back pain and other knock-on problems. The good news is that Pilates can help you to straighten your spine again and regain your maximum possible height.

Do you ever get twinges in your lower back?

Twinges in the lower back are the most common type of back pain in men, and it tends to occur in those who have protruding guts and weak abdominal muscles. There is supposed to be a natural curve in the lower back to help with shock absorption, but if it becomes pronounced you will develop lower back problems that could eventually lead to disc prolapse.

Known as lordosis, this pronounced curve in the lumbar spine causes the hip muscles to shorten, which then pulls the pelvis out of alignment. This curvature will ultimately lead to difficulty in walking if it is not addressed, preferably early on.

If you think you have lordosis, the Pilates solution is to work on strengthening the muscle groups of the central core – the abdominals, back extensors, glutes, hamstrings, pelvic floor and latissimus dorsi. This will pull the pelvis back into correct alignment and help to support your spine in its natural curves. In the meantime, take particular care when lifting or carrying anything remotely heavy.

Are there knots in your shoulders?

In the posture check in chapter 1, did you identify a forwards curve in your upper back? Does your chin jut outwards? And did you have trouble doing the plumbline challenge on pages 16–17? You may have a condition known as kyphosis, in which there is excessive forward curvature of the thoracic spine. This is not uncommon in very tall people who tend to stoop, or in those with desk jobs who spend a lot of time gazing at their computer screen, or those with driving jobs who sit hunched over the steering wheel.

If you have a forward-curving upper spine, you have to lift and jut your chin forwards to see where you are going. This can cause neck and shoulder tension, and will eventually cause breathing difficulties because the chest muscles are so tight that the ribs can't move in and out properly. You may also get lower back pain because when the weight of the upper body is leaning forwards, the lower spine needs to arch for you to keep your balance.

In Pilates, we relieve kyphosis by strengthening all the muscles of the upper and mid back, especially the latissimus dorsi and serratus anterior muscles. This helps to pull down the large diamond-shaped trapezius muscle that can get very bunched up in the shoulders, thus relieving tension in the neck.

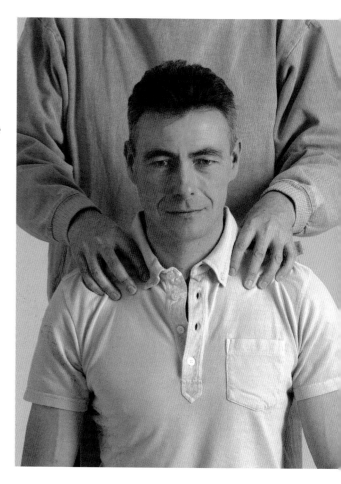

Are you asymmetrical?

We all have asymmetries in our bodies because the side we use most often will be strongest. However, if you identified anomalies during your posture check – such as one shoulder higher than the other, different-sized gaps between your lower arms and your hips or one hip bone lower than the other – it could mean that you have a condition called scoliosis. Here the spine curves to one side in the thoracic region and to the other side in the lumbar region, forming an 'S' shape.

This curvature can start in childhood if a child consistently carries a heavy schoolbag on one shoulder. It can result from having one leg longer than the other; or it can be the result of accidents or disease. Whatever the cause, it is progressive and can become seriously debilitating later in life if left unchecked.

Pilates can help to combat scoliosis, but because there are so many degrees of the condition and so many different patterns, you should consult a specialist first to get a clearer picture of what's going on with your spine. You should then book one-to-one Pilates lessons so an instructor can show you specifically how to strengthen some muscles groups and lengthen others to correct your particular kind of curvature.

How flexible is your spine?

Did you manage the tests on 3, 4, 6 and 8 in chapter 1? Your spine can lose its ability to rotate sideways or bend backwards or forwards through lack of muscle tone, shortening of the muscles on one or both sides due to poor posture or if the discs between vertebrae become compressed.

Disc compression in the lower back can lead to sciatica, a very painful condition in which the sciatic nerve, which runs from the pelvis through the buttocks and down into the legs, becomes trapped. Disc compression in the cervical spine can cause trapped nerves down the arms and pins and needles in the fingers, as well as nausea and breathlessness. Both of these disc compression conditions require medical advice, but strengthening the muscles of your back and abdomen will help to hold all the vertebrae in the correct position without collapsing on themselves.

A flexible spine is well worth working for. There are few things that make you look more elderly than being unable to pick up the post from the doormat without clutching your back. Your sports techniques will benefit from a strong, flexible back and you'll be better able to prevent injury.

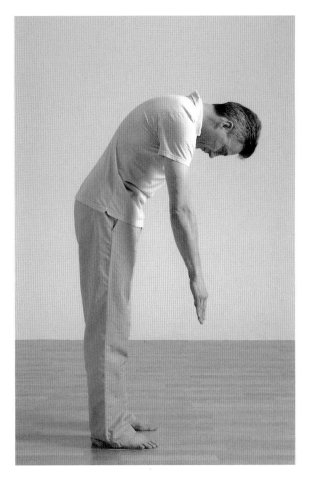

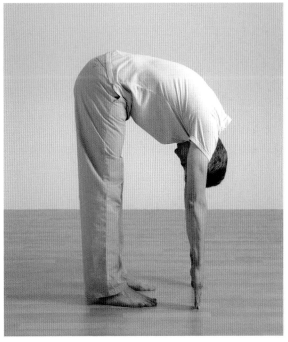

Do you have dodgy knees?

Knee problems seem to be endemic – almost as common as lower back pain. The knee is a complicated joint, held together by strong ligaments on either side and cruciate ligaments within – it needs good, balanced muscle tone in all the muscle groups round about to keep it stable. Problems are nearly always progressive, so don't put off getting medical advice. If your knee swells up every time you play tennis, it's trying to tell you something!

One cause of knee problems can be the pressure applied to the joint if your quadriceps muscles are much stronger than your hamstrings. This is why sprinters, who have very strong quads, are vulnerable to knee ligament injuries. Footballers and rugby players are even more at risk because of all that swerving and turning while running at speed.

Consistently sitting with your legs crossed can also cause knee problems. Most people tend to cross their legs the same way each time, so the muscles in one hip will shorten and tighten as a result, while the knee ligaments on the leg that you cross over are put under sideways pressure. And the rule is that consistently applying uneven pressure to any joint will lead to more wear and tear on it.

A simple ankle strain that makes you limp for a couple of weeks can cause knock-on effects in your knee, as can any foot problems that mean your weight is not being distributed evenly through that triangle shape described on page 18.

Lots of people don't walk correctly, either because of injuries or postural problems, or because they've just got into bad habits. To walk well, all the muscles in the legs, hips and buttocks need to work together. The ankles and feet need to move properly so that you can strike the ground with your heel first, roll through the foot, then push off with the toes. How did you manage the balance test on page 9? It's vital that you are using all your muscles in unison to be able to balance well.

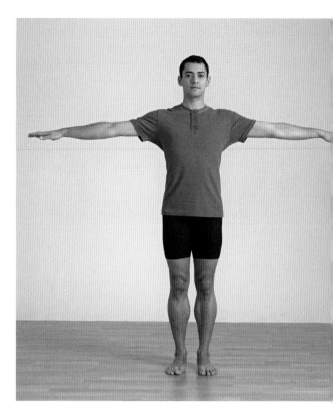

Do you have tight hamstrings?

Test 1 will have caught you out if this is your problem, and I doubt you will have been able to do the half squat in test 10. If your hamstrings are tight, you will feel a pulling on your lower back whenever you lean forwards, and you will start feeling twinges there before long. You will be shifting your pelvis out of the correct alignment, which means the spine is going to have to bend into unnatural curves to keep you balanced. Your hips won't be very mobile and you are likely to have knee problems as well.

If a piston ring breaks in a car, it damages the piston, and the connecting rod, and then the crankshaft and then your engine will seize up. The human body is constructed so that everything should work together like a well-tuned engine. If one bit is not working correctly, it puts strain on the rest and before you know it, you're flat on your back swallowing painkillers and watching daytime television.

Don't worry if you've identified tight hamstrings, though. Work through the routines in this book carefully and regularly and you'll see an improvement before long.

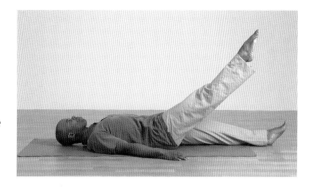

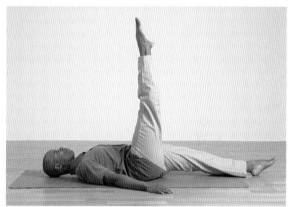

Are your shoulders even?

Or is one shoulder higher? I bet this is the side with which you use your computer mouse. And I bet it crunches when you massage into the shoulder muscle on that side.

Repetitive strain injury is also increasingly common for those who operate keyboards and it can be very debilitating, causing pain and weakness in the fingers, wrist, and arm on the affected side. If you are doing any kind of repetitive movement, it's important to make sure that your posture is good so that the workload is spread through the whole area rather than focused in one joint such as the wrist.

This advice also applies to musicians, dentists and anyone whose work involves repetitive actions (or those who spend their leisure time trying to get up to the next level on PlayStation). There are Pilates exercises that can help, but not if you carry on working with awkward postures.

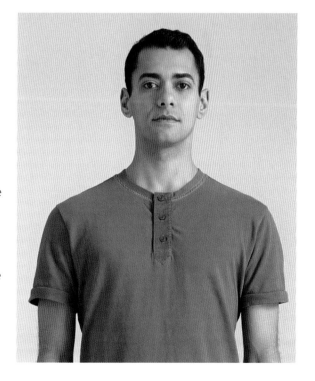

Are you overweight?

Sorry, but this had to come up. Lack of muscle tone in your abdomen can lead to lordosis, the lower back problem described on page 23 – and you are unlikely to have well-toned abdominal muscles if they are submerged beneath thick layers of fat. Obesity will also put extra strain on your hips, knees and ankles, and can prevent you from breathing fully and deeply.

There are various tests you can apply to judge whether you are carrying too much excess weight. The body mass index (BMI) is a weight-to-height ratio that is commonly used by doctors and health professionals. Just divide your weight in kilograms (stones) by the square of your height in metres (feet and inches):

$$weight \div [height \times height] = BMI$$

Check your score

Less than 15 Emaciated
15–19   Underweight
19–25   Fine
25–30   Overweight
Over 30 Obese

If you are a heavily muscled athlete you may get a high BMI reading even though you don't have much body fat. Your gym may have a set of bioelectrical impedance scales that measure body fat in relation to muscle mass, and men between the ages of 18 and 40 should ideally get a score of between 18 and 26 per cent body fat on these. Buy a set for your bathroom if you think it will motivate you to stay off the chips and lager.

Alternatively, there is a very simple measurement that seems to give a good indication of whether your weight is a problem or not, and that is your waist circumference. Research shows that if a man's waist circumference rises above 90 cm (35½ in), unhealthy metabolic changes start to take place; if it is above 100 cm (40 in), he is in a high-risk category for illnesses such as cardiovascular disease and Type 2 diabetes. Another telling body measurement is the waist-to-hip ratio (waist measurement ÷ hip measurement). This is regarded as high if it is above one. Fat stored in the gut is more harmful than fat stored anywhere else in the body, as it starts to act like an organ in its own right and release damaging chemicals into the bloodstream.

Pilates isn't an aerobic exercise system that can burn up body fat, but if you are on a weight-loss diet it will help to tone your muscles as they emerge from under the layers of fat so that you look and feel better more quickly. It will help make clothes look better on you and you should feel better about yourself.

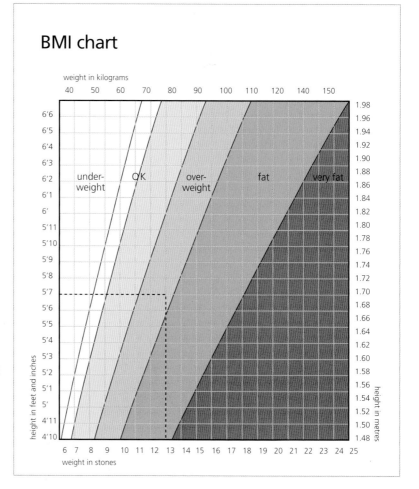

BMI chart

EVALUATING YOURSELF

Have you had an accident or an illness that has affected your body?

Poor posture is often the cause of imbalances in the body, but of course problems can also be caused by accidents or illness. If you are receiving treatment for an injury, talk to your specialist or physiotherapist before starting Pilates. Take this book and ask them to point out any exercises that could be especially useful for you, and any that you should avoid for the time being. Arthritis and osteoporosis both cause bone and joint problems and if you suffer from either, get advice from a specialist before starting Pilates.

It's important to learn to recognize the difference between an ache and a pain when you're exercising. An ache can usually be stretched out, but if you get a shooting pain that doesn't go away or that gets worse on movement, get it checked out. Stiffness can be worked through, but if it hurts when you try to move beyond a restricted range, seek advice. Clicks and crunches are not necessarily serious, but once again, check with your doctor if you're worried.

When did you last exercise?

If you haven't exercised since you were at school, you'll need to start very slowly. Don't try to move too quickly through the different phases of exercises described in chapters 3 and 4. Begin by concentrating on your posture, gently strengthening your core muscles, and walking around as much as possible during the day.

Don't launch into any new exercise regime with a macho attitude. If you race straight onto a hockey pitch or sign up for an off-piste skiing holiday when you haven't done anything more strenuous than carrying the rubbish out for the last six months, you're at serious risk of a heart attack or injury, or both.

If you've never done any Pilates before, you will find some of it tricky at first. This is no reflection on your abilities. Olympic athletes would find some aspects of Pilates difficult because their training probably wouldn't have the same emphasis on flexibility. There's a lot to remember when you start Pilates because you have to coordinate your breathing with several different muscle movements, and you have to concentrate hard to make sure you move the correct muscles and not others.

Don't rush through the programmes in this book – it's not a race. The quality of your movement is crucial, and if you are not in exactly the right alignment the exercise will be much less effective. It's much better to do one perfect hip roll than 20 sloppy static abs! You'll get the idea as we go along.

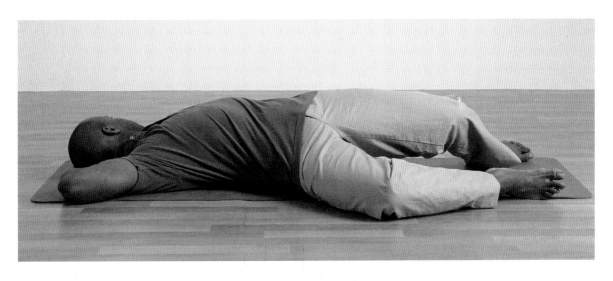

Chapter 3
The posture workout

These won't be the toughest exercises you've ever tried, but they are vital to help you get the correct muscle groups working. Mastering these simpler movements now will save you from imbalance, tension and injury later on in the programme. Pilates exercises are very precise, so take care when adopting the starting position to make sure you are exactly aligned, and follow all instructions to the letter. Don't race through them: move slowly and smoothly, ensuring that you can feel the correct muscles doing the work.

Wear loose, comfortable clothing and socks, or have bare feet, but no shoes or trainers. The only 'equipment' you'll need is a few cushions or pillows, a small towel, a rug or mat to lie on and a chair or stool without arms. Good luck!

Static abs

Area they work
- Abdominals.

Points to watch
- Breathe in through your nose and out through your mouth in all Pilates exercises.
- Don't squeeze the cushion or towel between your knees.
- Keep chest and shoulders relaxed into the floor.
- Maintain the correct spinal alignment; don't press your lower back down to the floor.

Contraindications
- If you have lordosis, place a pillow under your upper back as you perform this abdominal exercise.

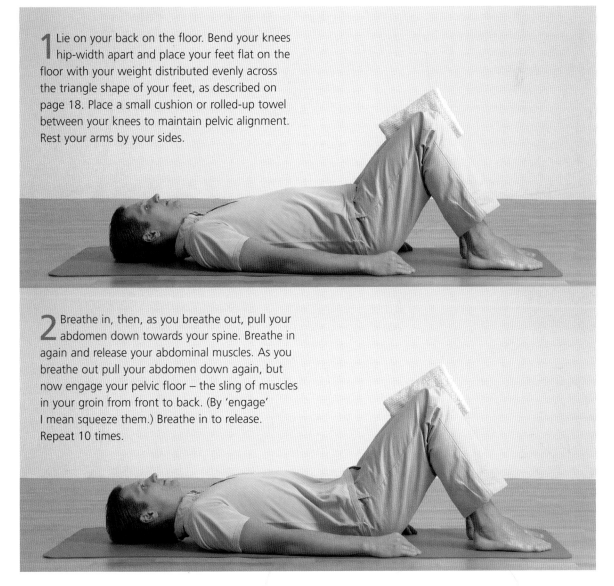

1 Lie on your back on the floor. Bend your knees hip-width apart and place your feet flat on the floor with your weight distributed evenly across the triangle shape of your feet, as described on page 18. Place a small cushion or rolled-up towel between your knees to maintain pelvic alignment. Rest your arms by your sides.

2 Breathe in, then, as you breathe out, pull your abdomen down towards your spine. Breathe in again and release your abdominal muscles. As you breathe out pull your abdomen down again, but now engage your pelvic floor – the sling of muscles in your groin from front to back. (By 'engage' I mean squeeze them.) Breathe in to release. Repeat 10 times.

Bridging

Areas it works

- Abdominals, pelvis, lower back, hamstrings, glutes.

Points to watch

- Make sure your abdominal muscles are engaged before lifting upwards.
- Keep your waist long; don't allow the spine to curl.
- Keep neck and shoulders relaxed into the floor.
- Don't squeeze the towel between your thighs.
- Movements should be slow and controlled, not jerky.
- Breathe in through your nose and out through your mouth.

Contraindications

- Stop immediately if you feel any lower back pain when doing this, as it means your abdominals are not yet strong enough to protect the lumbar spine. Focus on doing abdominal exercises then try again in a week or so.

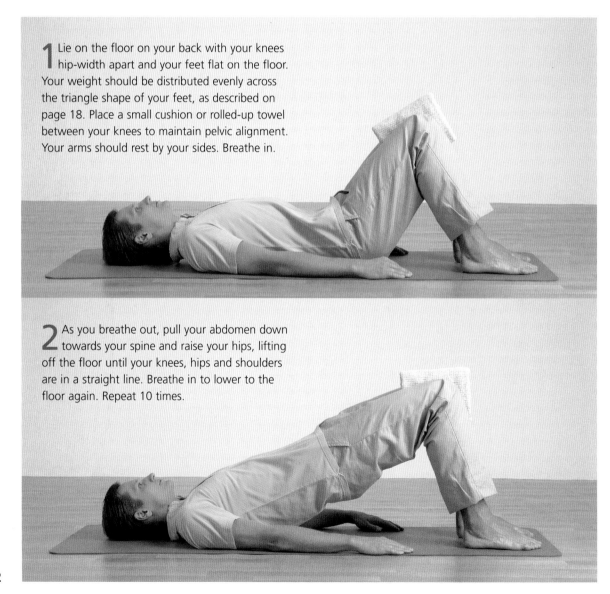

1 Lie on the floor on your back with your knees hip-width apart and your feet flat on the floor. Your weight should be distributed evenly across the triangle shape of your feet, as described on page 18. Place a small cushion or rolled-up towel between your knees to maintain pelvic alignment. Your arms should rest by your sides. Breathe in.

2 As you breathe out, pull your abdomen down towards your spine and raise your hips, lifting off the floor until your knees, hips and shoulders are in a straight line. Breathe in to lower to the floor again. Repeat 10 times.

Leg slides

Areas they work
- Abdominals, pelvic, legs area.

Points to watch
- Don't let your pelvis move; keep the hips level. If your pelvis does move, stop and return to this exercise later when your pelvis is more stable. You could try practising with the leg and the arm moving separately.
- Your shoulder joint may restrict the movement, but don't try to force it; keep within a comfortable range.
- Keep your abdominals engaged throughout to support the lumbar spine.
- Feel your abdominal and leg muscles working together.

Contraindications
- Stop immediately if you feel any pain in your lower back or shoulders.

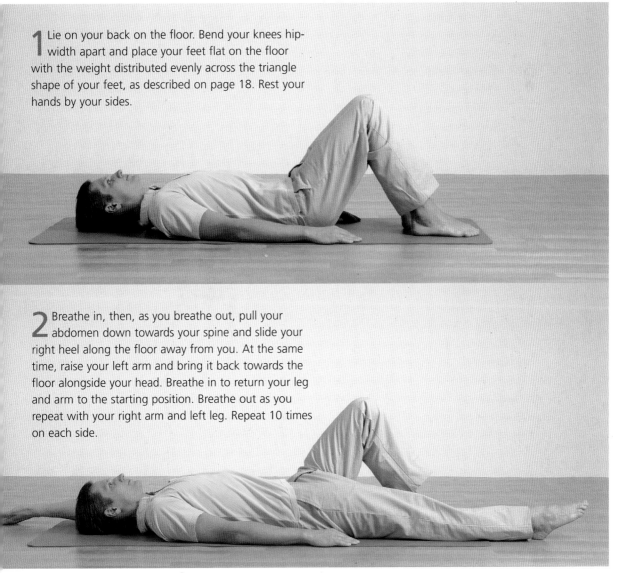

1 Lie on your back on the floor. Bend your knees hip-width apart and place your feet flat on the floor with the weight distributed evenly across the triangle shape of your feet, as described on page 18. Rest your hands by your sides.

2 Breathe in, then, as you breathe out, pull your abdomen down towards your spine and slide your right heel along the floor away from you. At the same time, raise your left arm and bring it back towards the floor alongside your head. Breathe in to return your leg and arm to the starting position. Breathe out as you repeat with your right arm and left leg. Repeat 10 times on each side.

Dip and stretch

Areas it works

- Abdominals, multifidous (in lower back).

Points to watch

- Make sure your abdominal muscles are engaged throughout and that you can feel your lower abdominal muscles doing the work.
- As the leg straightens, you should almost feel your spine lengthening away from it.
- Keep your pelvis stable; avoid leaning into the hip on the side that is moving. Imagine that there is a ruler placed across from hip bone to hip bone and that you have to keep it level as you work.

Contraindications

- Stop immediately if you feel any lower back pain.

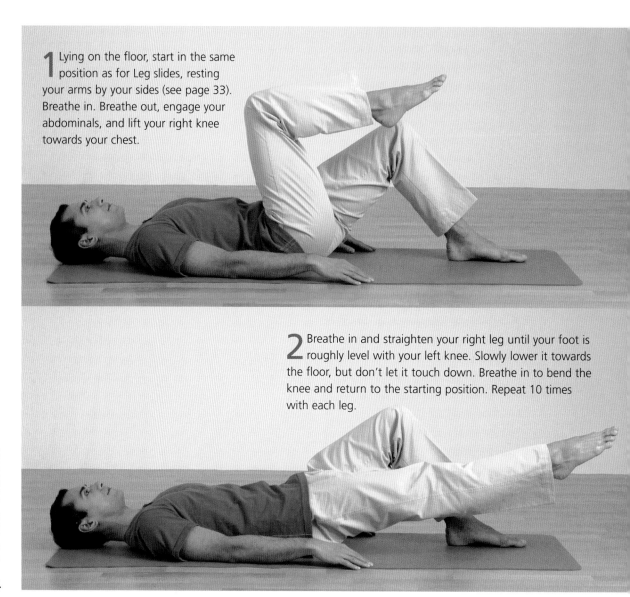

1 Lying on the floor, start in the same position as for Leg slides, resting your arms by your sides (see page 33). Breathe in. Breathe out, engage your abdominals, and lift your right knee towards your chest.

2 Breathe in and straighten your right leg until your foot is roughly level with your left knee. Slowly lower it towards the floor, but don't let it touch down. Breathe in to bend the knee and return to the starting position. Repeat 10 times with each leg.

Glute squeezes

Area they work
- Gluteus maximus (buttocks).

Points to watch
- Don't let your legs rotate inwards.
- It's not a massive clenching movement – just a firm squeeze.
- If one buttock feels stronger than the other, try starting the squeeze with the weaker one and they should soon even up.
- Avoid over-using your abdominals; this exercise is all about the glutes.

Contraindications
- If you have different leg lengths, or instability in your lower back, lie face down on the floor to do this exercise. Place a pillow under your hips and another one under your forehead.

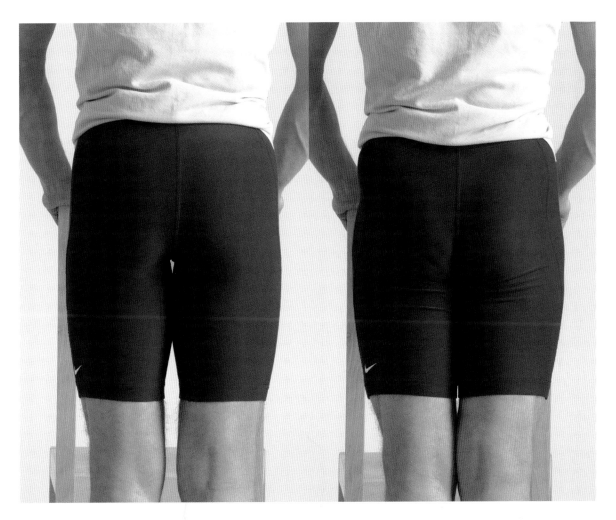

1 Stand up straight with your hands resting on the back of a chair or against a wall. Your feet should be together.

2 Breathe out, squeeze your sitting bones together and downwards, and engage your abdominals. Don't let your legs rotate outwards. Hold for 5 seconds. Breathe in to relax and repeat 10 times.

Hamstring curls

Areas they work
• Hamstrings, glutes.

Points to watch
• Make sure you keep your leg moving in a straight line so the knee is in alignment throughout.

• Remember to breathe in through your nose and out through your mouth. I'm going to stop reminding you about this from now on, but don't forget as it is an important part of the exercises in this book.

Contraindications
• If you have knee problems, it can help to place a rolled-up towel under the thigh, just above the knees, so the kneecaps are not pressing down on the floor.

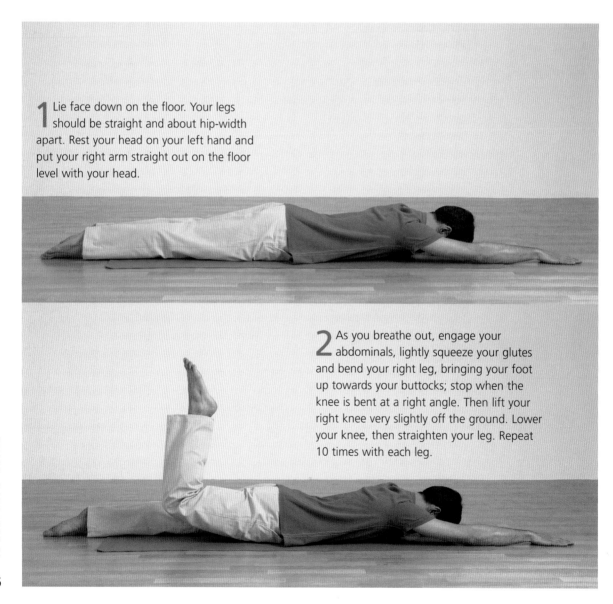

1 Lie face down on the floor. Your legs should be straight and about hip-width apart. Rest your head on your left hand and put your right arm straight out on the floor level with your head.

2 As you breathe out, engage your abdominals, lightly squeeze your glutes and bend your right leg, bringing your foot up towards your buttocks; stop when the knee is bent at a right angle. Then lift your right knee very slightly off the ground. Lower your knee, then straighten your leg. Repeat 10 times with each leg.

The Cobra (1)

Areas it works

- Latissimus dorsi muscles, lower back, abdominals (stretch).

Points to watch

- Don't push yourself up with your arms; you should be able to feel the latissimus dorsi muscles just beneath your shoulderblades doing the work.
- Keep your hip bones on the floor.
- There's a more advanced version of The Cobra on page 124.

Contraindications

- If your lower back feels uncomfortable, keep the movement small and gradually increase the lift each time you try it.

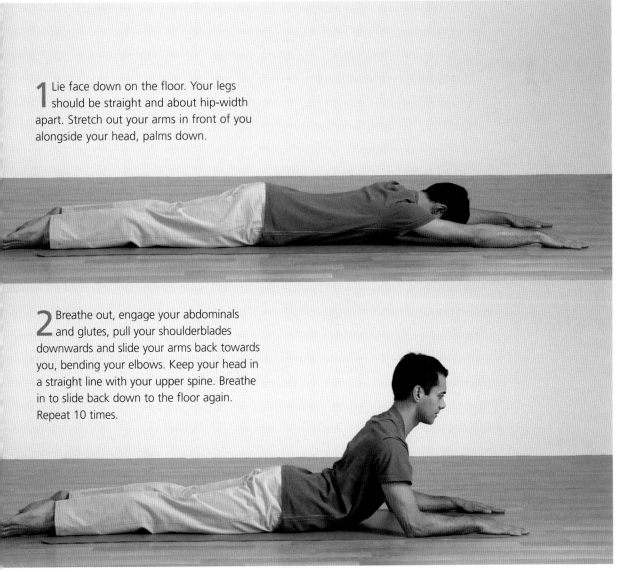

1 Lie face down on the floor. Your legs should be straight and about hip-width apart. Stretch out your arms in front of you alongside your head, palms down.

2 Breathe out, engage your abdominals and glutes, pull your shoulderblades downwards and slide your arms back towards you, bending your elbows. Keep your head in a straight line with your upper spine. Breathe in to slide back down to the floor again. Repeat 10 times.

The Arrow

Area it works
- Latissimus dorsi muscles.

Points to watch
- Don't let your head lead the backwards movement; your upper spine should remain in a straight line. Think of lengthening your head away from your body.
- Make sure your abdominals are engaged throughout.

Contraindications
- Try this very carefully if you have lower back problems and stop if you feel any twinges in your back.
- If you have trouble drawing your shoulderblades down the back, keep practising The Cobra and the other upper back exercises in this chapter.

1 Lie face down on the floor with your legs straight and hip-width apart. Rest your arms by your sides. Breathe in.

2 As you breathe out, engage your abdominals and glutes and let your arms lift until they are roughly in line with your hips. Draw your shoulderblades down and lift your breastbone – your upper body will lift upwards. Hold for 5 seconds. Breathe in as you lower your arms and upper body to the floor. Repeat 10 times.

Adductors

Area they work
- Abdominals, adductor muscles (inner thighs).

Points to watch
- You should be able to feel the inner thigh muscles working on the leg you are sliding across.
- Use a hand to push down hard on your opposite hip to prevent it lifting as you move the leg.
- Keep your leg straight, but without tension.

Contraindications
- If you have tight hamstrings, stretch them before you do this exercise. There are some hamstring stretches on pages 120–21.

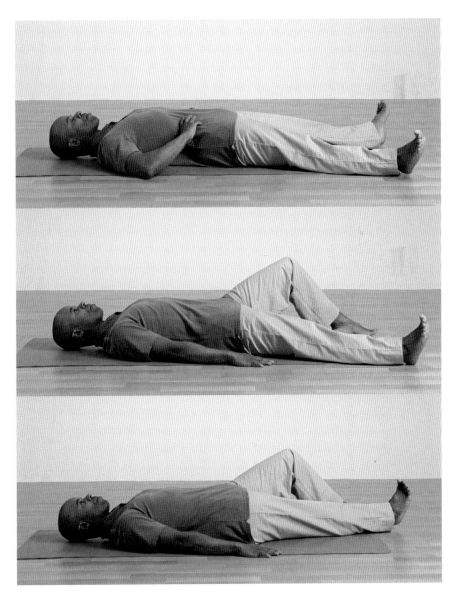

1 Lie on the floor on your back and place your hands on your hips. Extend your legs in a 'V' shape.

2 Bend your left knee and place the left foot on the ground. Relax your right arm onto the floor. Rotate your right leg outwards very slightly.

3 As you breathe out, engage your abdominals and slide your right leg as far as you can towards your left foot without lifting it off the floor. Breathe in to slide it back to the starting position. Repeat 10 times with each leg.

Back stretch (1)

Area it works

• Lower back.

Points to watch

• When getting into the starting position, don't lift both knees to your chest at the same time. Lift one and then the other. When you've finished, lower them one at a time.

• Keep your elbows wide and shoulders relaxed into the floor.

Contraindications

• Be wary of this stretch if you have restricted hip movement or have had a hip replacement.

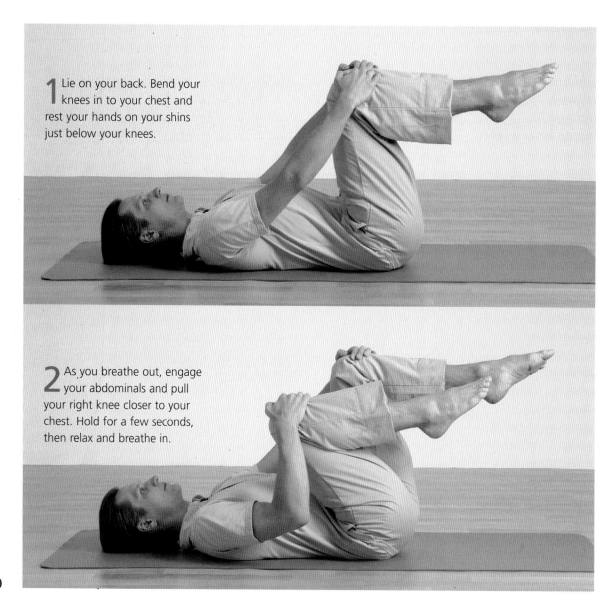

1 Lie on your back. Bend your knees in to your chest and rest your hands on your shins just below your knees.

2 As you breathe out, engage your abdominals and pull your right knee closer to your chest. Hold for a few seconds, then relax and breathe in.

BACK STRETCH

40

3 Next, as you breathe out, pull your left knee closer to your chest, then relax and breathe in.

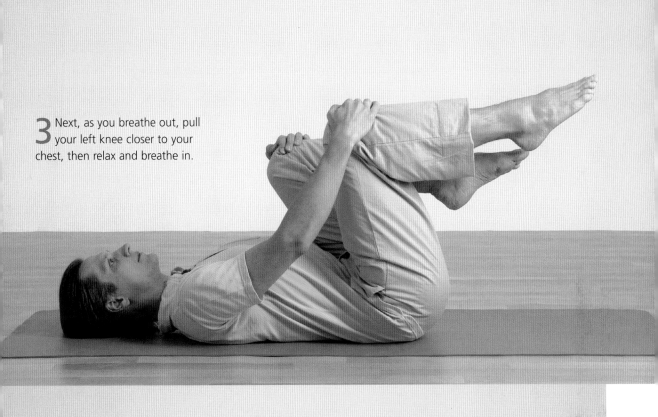

4 Now, as you breathe out, pull both knees together to your chest, then relax and breathe in. Hold your knees and feet together and then circle them slowly (4 times) clockwise and (4 times) anticlockwise, as if you are drawing circles on a blackboard directly above you. Breathe easily throughout. Repeat 4 times.

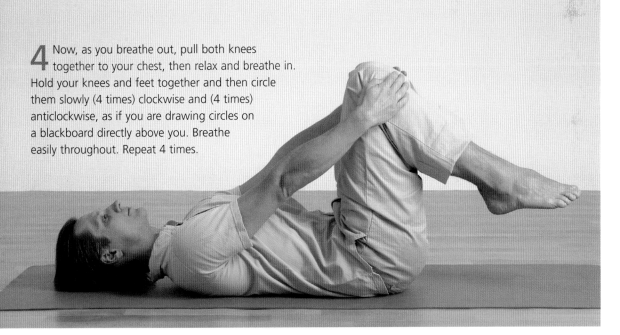

Hip rolls (1)

Area they work
- Abdominals, mainly the oblique muscles.

Points to watch
- Use your abdominals rather than your leg muscles to control the movements of your knees. If you think about the muscles working, this can actually help to activate them.
- You can get a bigger stretch down the side by letting your hip rise off the floor in step 2.

Contraindications
- If you have excessive lordosis, try placing your feet on a low stool or table for this exercise.
- Don't try this exercise at all if you have lower back injuries, a hip replacement or knee injuries.

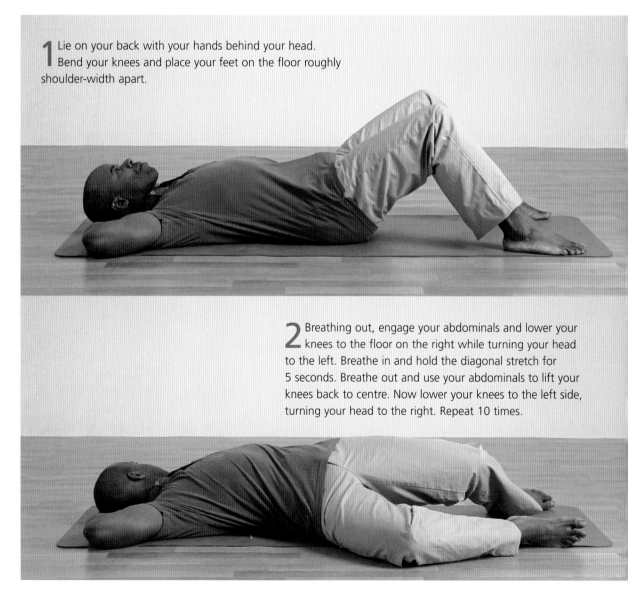

1 Lie on your back with your hands behind your head. Bend your knees and place your feet on the floor roughly shoulder-width apart.

2 Breathing out, engage your abdominals and lower your knees to the floor on the right while turning your head to the left. Breathe in and hold the diagonal stretch for 5 seconds. Breathe out and use your abdominals to lift your knees back to centre. Now lower your knees to the left side, turning your head to the right. Repeat 10 times.

The 90:90

Area it works
• Lower abdominals.

Points to watch
• It's a very small movement; your tailbone should lift no more than 2 cm (¾ in).
• You should be able to feel this working deep in the lower abdominal muscles.
• Your lower legs shouldn't lift or move around – keep them parallel to the floor.

Contraindications
• If you can't manage The 90:90 at first, do the same exercise with your lower legs resting on a chair so that your hips and knees are bent at right angles.

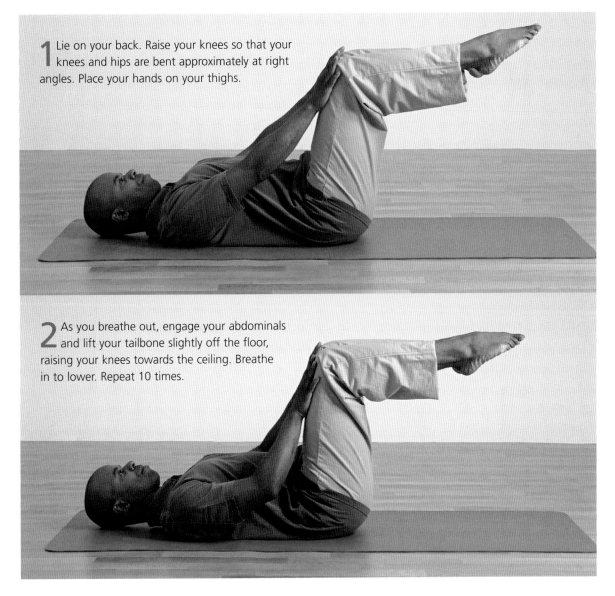

1 Lie on your back. Raise your knees so that your knees and hips are bent approximately at right angles. Place your hands on your thighs.

2 As you breathe out, engage your abdominals and lift your tailbone slightly off the floor, raising your knees towards the ceiling. Breathe in to lower. Repeat 10 times.

Shoulder shrugs

Areas they work

- Trapezius, latissimus dorsi muscles.

Points to watch

- Don't hunch your shoulders up tightly.
- Concentrate hard on drawing down the latissimus dorsi muscles beneath your shoulderblades in step 2. It may seem like a very simple exercise, but to master this action it is important to be precise.

Contraindications

- Only those with very serious neck problems would have trouble with this.

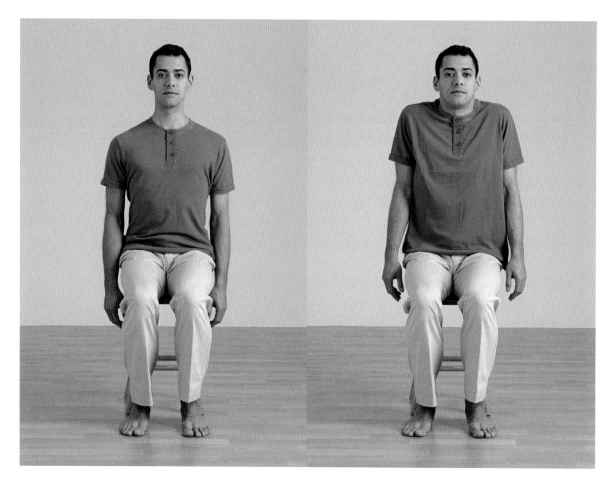

1 Sit on a chair without arms, or a stool, at the correct height so that your hips and knees are bent at right angles. Let your arms hang by your sides.

2 Shrug your shoulders up to your ears. Then slide your shoulderblades down your back to bring your shoulders back to the starting position. Repeat 10 times.

Sitting lats

Areas they work
- Latissimus dorsi muscles, trapezius.

Points to watch
- Keep your shoulders down throughout this exercise and use the latissimus dorsi muscles to control the movement.
- Stop your shoulders from curling forwards.
- Try to feel your chest opening out as you move your arms behind you.
- Keep your eyeline up and your spine long.

Contraindications
- If you feel any strain in your neck or shoulders, you are doing this exercise incorrectly. Keep practising Shoulder shrugs (see page 44), Arm openings (see page 46) and The Cobra (see page 37) to learn how to activate and loosen the thoracic spine.

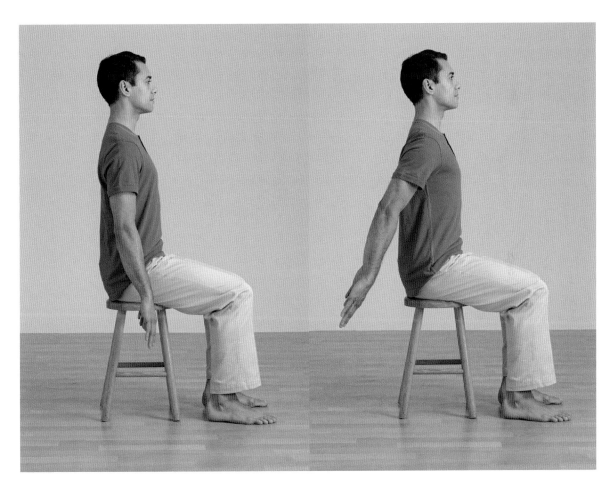

1 Sit on a chair without arms, or a stool, at the correct height so that your hips and knees are bent at right angles. Let your arms hang by your sides.

2 As you breathe out, engage your abdominals, slide your shoulderblades down and push your right palm backwards against the air. Breathe in to bring your right arm forwards again. Repeat 10 times with each arm, then breathe out and push both palms back together. Breathe in to bring them forwards. Repeat 10 times.

Arm openings

Areas they work

- All the muscles round the shoulder joints and shoulderblades.

Points to watch

- Leave a slight gap between your elbows and your waist.
- You shouldn't feel any tension in your neck or shoulders; if you do, stop and try again when your upper back is looser.
- During the movement, your upper arms will rotate and your chest will open out, but you should feel the latissimus dorsi muscles in your mid back doing the work.

Contraindications

- Those with tennis elbow or any kind of shoulder impingement could have a problem with this exercise.

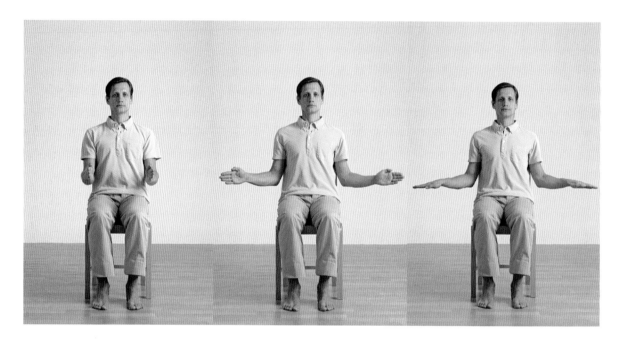

1 Sit on a stool or chair without arms. Bend your elbows at right angles and position them slightly forwards from your shoulders, with the palms facing each other. Check that your shoulders are relaxed.

2 As you breathe in, engage your abdominals and open your arms outwards, keeping your elbows in the same position like a pivot. Breathe out to bring your arms back to the starting position. Repeat 10 times.

3 Next, turn your palms to face upwards and repeat the opening movement 10 times. Turn your palms downwards and repeat 10 times.

The Cossack

Areas it works
- Mobilizes the mid back and thoracic spine.

Points to watch
- Don't let your shoulders do the work – keep them relaxed.
- Keep your spine straight and imagine your upper body rotating around it.
- Keep your hips and knees absolutely still.
- It may help if you place a pole of some kind across your back and through the gap between your elbows and ribs on either side – see Twisting with a pole on page 85.

Contraindications
- Avoid excessive twisting if your lower back is at all vulnerable.
- If you have restricted movement in your shoulders, grasp the forearms in front of your body instead and turn that way.

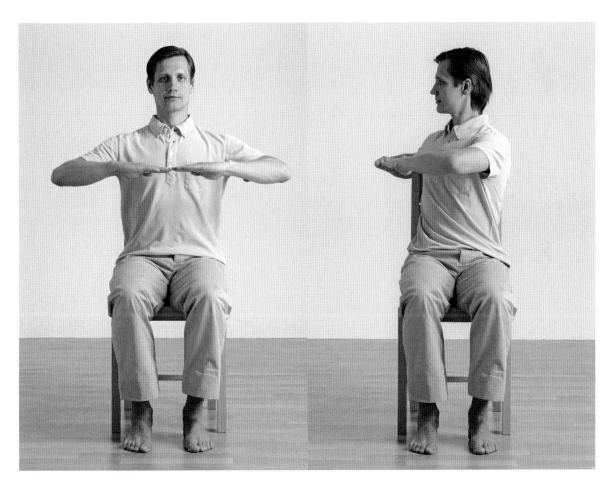

1 Sit on a stool or chair without arms. Bend your elbows and touch your fingertips together in front of your breastbone. Breathe in.

2 As you breathe out, engage your abdominals, slide your shoulderblades down and turn your upper body to the right. Go back as far as you can. Breathe in to return to centre. Then, breathe out to turn your upper body to the left. Repeat 10 times in each direction.

Chapter 4
Moving forwards

This chapter includes two workouts: Intermediate (pages 49–59) and Advanced (pages 60–73). Neither of them is easy. For both sets of exercises, it is important to remember the posture lessons you learned in the last chapter and to use them to help you attain the correct positions and perform the movements in a precise and controlled manner. If you find an exercise difficult, leave it for now and try again in a week or so when you are stronger and more flexible. Never persevere if anything hurts.

Be aware that there are no specific contraindications noted in the Advanced workout, because if you have any problems with your joints, back or neck, you shouldn't attempt these exercises at all. And even if you don't have any aches and pains, you must be able to perform all the exercises in the Intermediate workout smoothly before you move on to this section. You won't be able to do them accurately unless your core stability is very strong.

The Hundred (1)

Areas it works
- Abdominals, arms, shoulders, stamina.

Points to watch
- Don't lift with your neck; make sure your whole upper body curls forwards.
- Keep your abdominals engaged at all times or you risk straining your lower back.
- Pull your abdominals further in each time you breathe out.
- Hold your torso in a 'C' shape rather than a 'V'.

Contraindications
- If you have lower back problems, you may not be able to do this exercise until your core stability is stronger. Stop if you feel any strain.

1 Lie on your back and raise your knees so your thighs are bent at right angles above your hips. Keep your knees, thighs and feet together. Place your hands just below the knees. Keep your elbows wide and your shoulders relaxed into the floor.

2 Breathe out, engage your abdominals and use your hands to help lift your upper body from the floor.

3 Engage your glutes and thigh muscles and lower your legs slightly until your thighs are at an angle of 80 degrees to the floor. Stretch your arms down by your sides at hip level. Pump your arms up and down without touching the floor, while you breathe in for 5 counts and out for 5 counts, until you have pumped your arms 100 times. Then lower your upper body and then your feet to the floor.

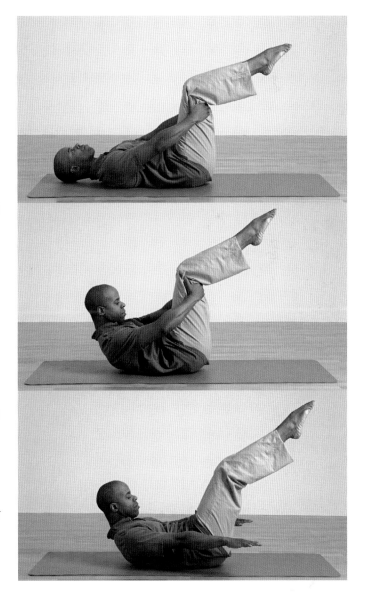

Roll-ups

Areas they work
- Abdominals, stretches spine and hamstrings.

Points to watch
- Keep your hips and legs still as you roll up and down. Squeezing your inner thighs together will help.
- Think of stretching and lengthening your spine. Keep your shoulders down and relaxed throughout.
- If you find it difficult to control the roll-back, try doing it with bent knees.

Contraindications
- Take care if you suffer with lower back or hamstring problems.

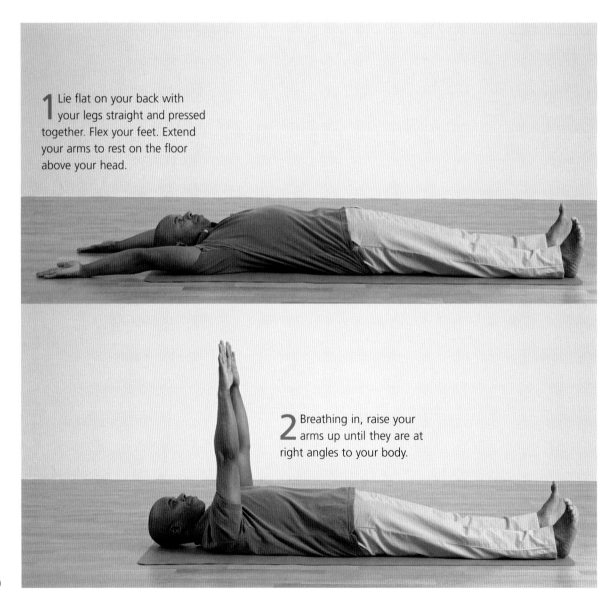

1 Lie flat on your back with your legs straight and pressed together. Flex your feet. Extend your arms to rest on the floor above your head.

2 Breathing in, raise your arms up until they are at right angles to your body.

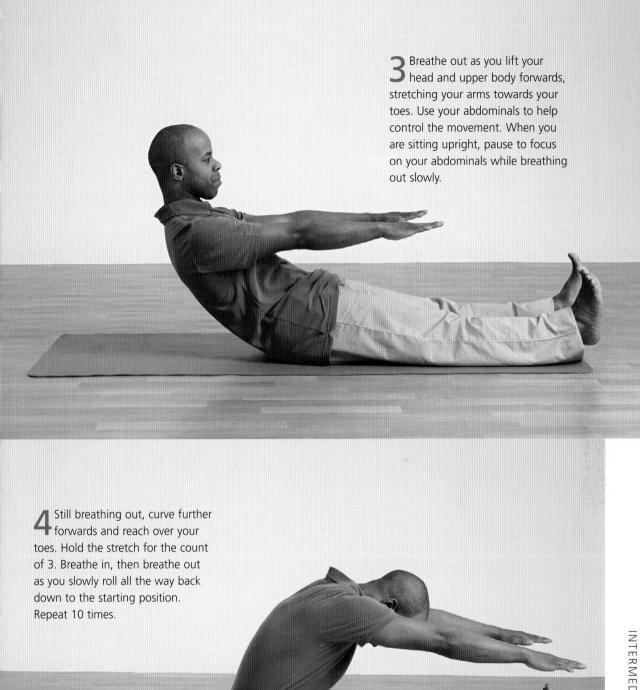

3 Breathe out as you lift your head and upper body forwards, stretching your arms towards your toes. Use your abdominals to help control the movement. When you are sitting upright, pause to focus on your abdominals while breathing out slowly.

4 Still breathing out, curve further forwards and reach over your toes. Hold the stretch for the count of 3. Breathe in, then breathe out as you slowly roll all the way back down to the starting position. Repeat 10 times.

Criss-cross

Areas it works
- Abdominals, especially oblique muscles.

Points to watch
- Don't twist with your shoulder – lift the entire upper body and twist from the waist.
- Use your glutes to keep the outstretched leg at an angle of roughly 45 degrees to the floor. The exercise will be much harder if it sinks too low down.
- Keep your hips stable throughout.

Contraindications
- Approach this with caution if you have lower back or neck problems.

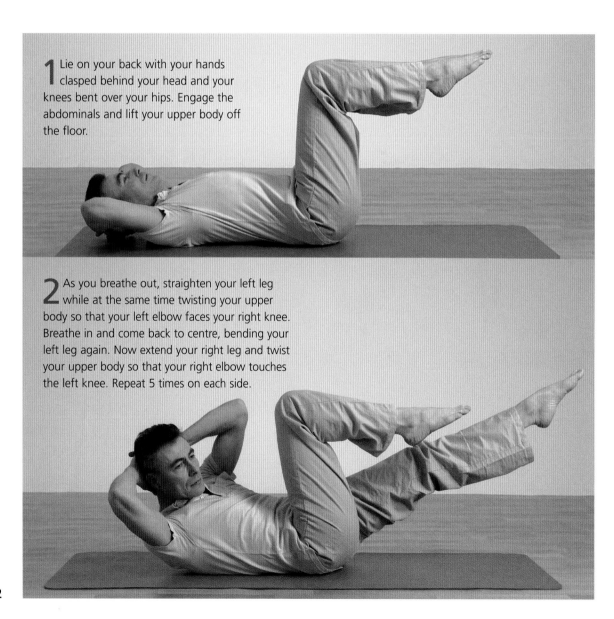

1 Lie on your back with your hands clasped behind your head and your knees bent over your hips. Engage the abdominals and lift your upper body off the floor.

2 As you breathe out, straighten your left leg while at the same time twisting your upper body so that your left elbow faces your right knee. Breathe in and come back to centre, bending your left leg again. Now extend your right leg and twist your upper body so that your right elbow touches the left knee. Repeat 5 times on each side.

Rolling like a ball

Areas it works
• Balance, spine massage.

Points to watch
• Pull your abdominals to your spine throughout to protect your back and neck.
• Keep your head tucked in at all times.
• Keep your shoulders relaxed.

Contraindications
• Be wary of this exercise if you have any spinal or back problems.

1 Sit on the floor with your knees bent up to your chest. Hold your ankles in your hands so that you are balanced on your tailbone. Tuck your head down so that you can imagine you are making a circular shape, like a ball.

2 Engage your abdominals and use this movement to initiate a rocking motion without letting your feet touch the floor. Roll back.

3 Squeeze your heels towards your buttocks to come forwards. Breathe in as you roll back and breathe out as you come up again. Develop a rhythm. Repeat 10 times.

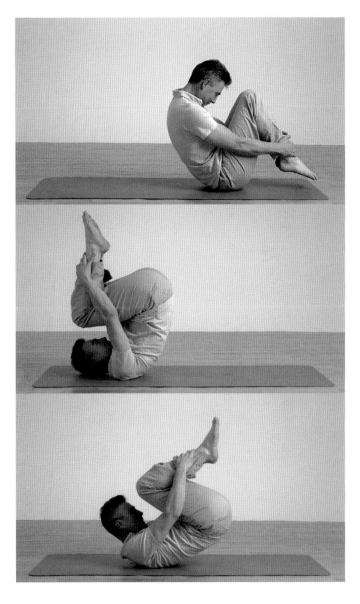

Double leg side lifts

Areas they work
- Oblique muscles, quadratus lumborum.

Points to watch
- Keep your heels, tailbone and neck in line as you lift.
- Use your abdominals, inner thighs and glutes to control the movement and protect your lower back.
- Don't let your neck tense – turn it slightly towards the floor as you lift.

Contraindications
- If you have lower back problems, you may not be able to do this exercise until you have built up your core stability.

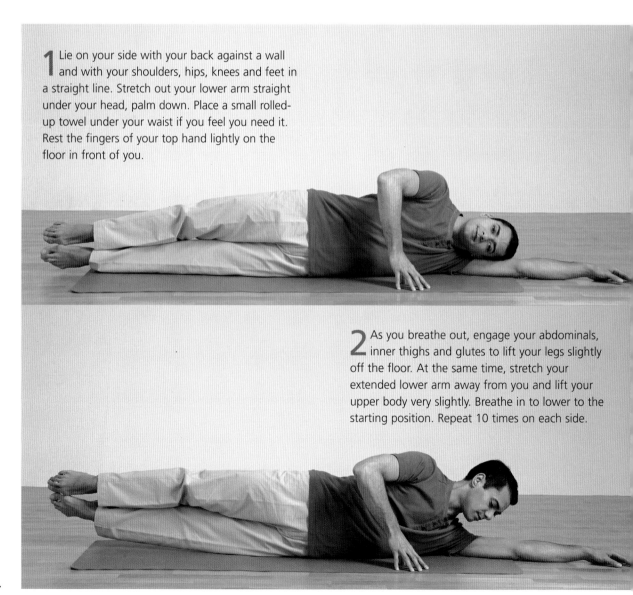

1 Lie on your side with your back against a wall and with your shoulders, hips, knees and feet in a straight line. Stretch out your lower arm straight under your head, palm down. Place a small rolled-up towel under your waist if you feel you need it. Rest the fingers of your top hand lightly on the floor in front of you.

2 As you breathe out, engage your abdominals, inner thighs and glutes to lift your legs slightly off the floor. At the same time, stretch your extended lower arm away from you and lift your upper body very slightly. Breathe in to lower to the starting position. Repeat 10 times on each side.

Swimming

Area it works
- Lower back.

Points to watch
- Keep your abdominals strongly engaged to protect your lower back.
- Raise the arm and leg to the same height – not more than 12 cm (4½ in) off the floor.
- Keep your shoulders down and relaxed; lift rather than stretch your arms.

Contraindications
- Stop if you feel any lower back discomfort and try again when your abdominals are stronger.

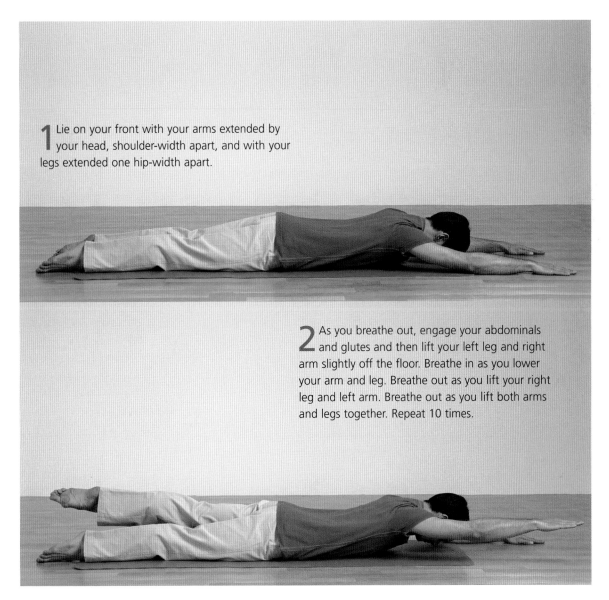

1 Lie on your front with your arms extended by your head, shoulder-width apart, and with your legs extended one hip-width apart.

2 As you breathe out, engage your abdominals and glutes and then lift your left leg and right arm slightly off the floor. Breathe in as you lower your arm and leg. Breathe out as you lift your right leg and left arm. Breathe out as you lift both arms and legs together. Repeat 10 times.

Leg pull-ups

Areas they work

- Glutes, hamstrings, arms, shoulders.

Points to watch

- Keep your hips lifted off the mat and your abdominals engaged throughout.
- Don't sink your weight into your arms or shoulders.

Contraindications

- Be careful if you suffer with wrist, elbow or shoulder problems.

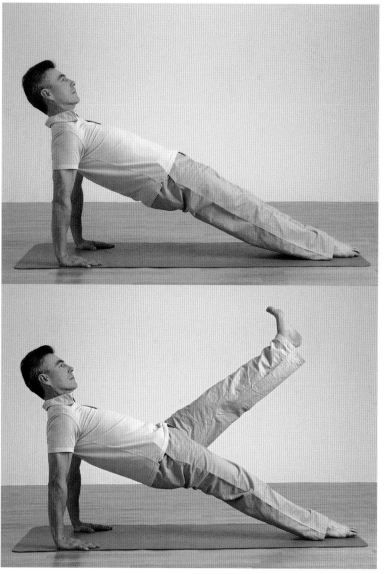

1 Sit on a mat on the floor with your legs straight out in front of you. Rest your palms on the floor by your sides with your fingers pointing towards your feet. Press down into your hands to lift your hips off the mat. Balance in this position with your legs straight and pressed together, toes pointing.

2 Breathe in and kick one leg as high as you can without losing your balance. At the top of the kick, flex your foot, then breathe out as you lower it again, stretching through the heel. As it gets close to the floor, but just before it touches, point your toe and kick up again, breathing in. Repeat 3 times with each leg.

Spine stretch

Areas it works
• Hamstrings, spine.

Points to watch
• Keep the 'C' shape in your spine and avoid stretching forwards from the hips.
• Keep your shoulders down and relaxed, away from your ears.
• Use your abdominals as you gradually roll back up, lifting your head last.
• Don't let your legs turn inwards.

Contraindications
• Don't try this if you have osteoporosis.

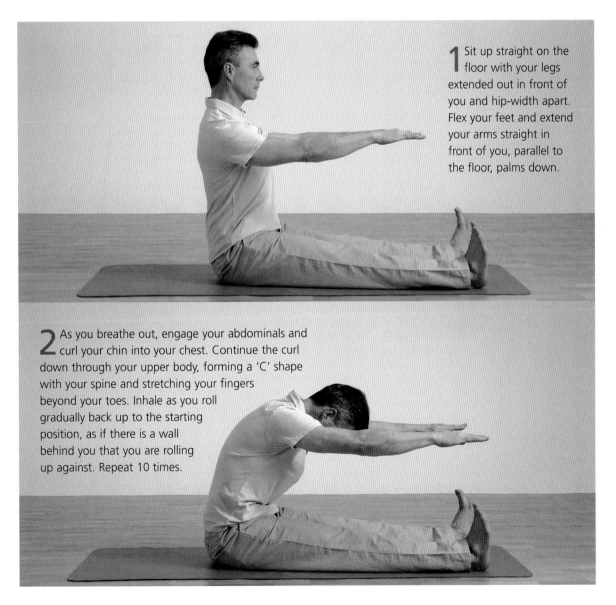

1 Sit up straight on the floor with your legs extended out in front of you and hip-width apart. Flex your feet and extend your arms straight in front of you, parallel to the floor, palms down.

2 As you breathe out, engage your abdominals and curl your chin into your chest. Continue the curl down through your upper body, forming a 'C' shape with your spine and stretching your fingers beyond your toes. Inhale as you roll gradually back up to the starting position, as if there is a wall behind you that you are rolling up against. Repeat 10 times.

Rowing (1)

Areas it works
- Abdominals, back, hamstrings.

Points to watch
- Keep your spine and waist long and your feet flexed throughout this exercise.
- Keep your shoulders down while your arms are over your head.

Contraindications
- Take care if you have lower back problems or any shoulder impingement.

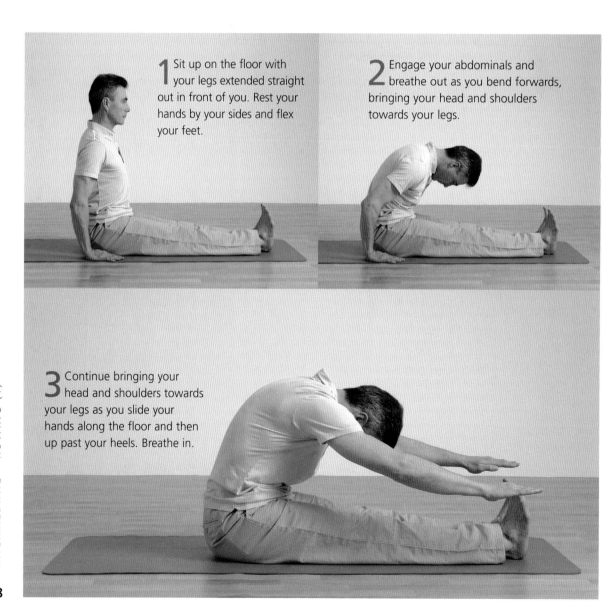

1 Sit up on the floor with your legs extended straight out in front of you. Rest your hands by your sides and flex your feet.

2 Engage your abdominals and breathe out as you bend forwards, bringing your head and shoulders towards your legs.

3 Continue bringing your head and shoulders towards your legs as you slide your hands along the floor and then up past your heels. Breathe in.

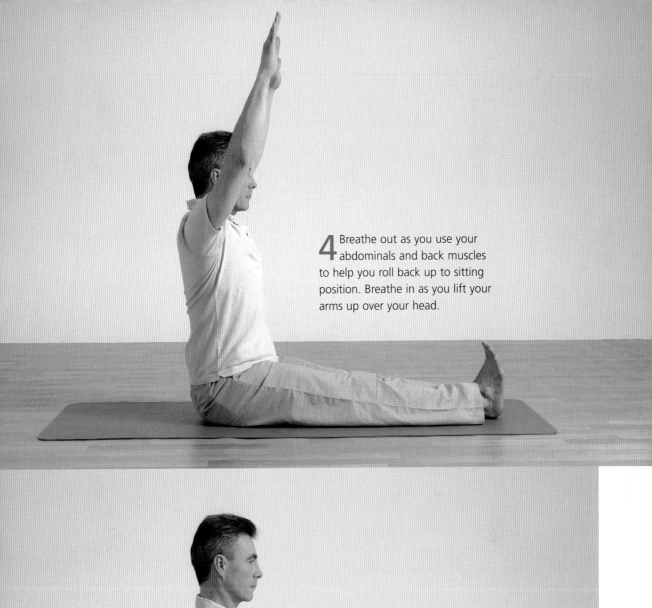

4 Breathe out as you use your abdominals and back muscles to help you roll back up to sitting position. Breathe in as you lift your arms up over your head.

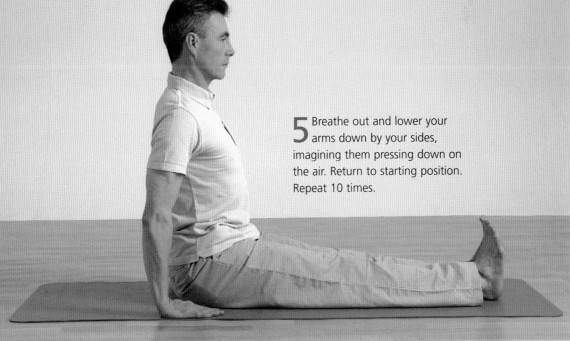

5 Breathe out and lower your arms down by your sides, imagining them pressing down on the air. Return to starting position. Repeat 10 times.

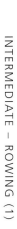

The Hundred (2)

Areas it works

- Abdominals, stamina.

Points to watch

- Don't lower your legs further than you can manage without your back arching.
- Keep your abdominals strong and watch that you can't feel any tension in the neck.
- If you have trouble with this version, go back to stage 1 of The Hundred on page 49 and try stage 2 again when your abdominals are stronger.

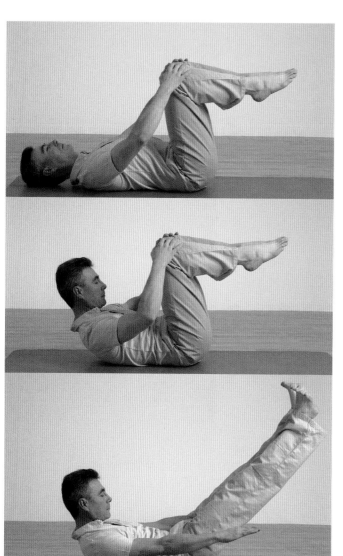

1 Lie on your back and raise your knees so they are bent at right angles above your hips, with thighs, knees and feet touching. Place your hands just below the knees. Keep your elbows wide and your shoulders relaxed into the floor.

2 Breathe out, engage your abdominals and use your hands to help lift your upper body from the floor.

3 Engage your glutes and thigh muscles and stretch your arms down by your sides at hip level. Straighten your legs so that they are at an angle of approximately 60 degrees to the floor, with your feet flexed and turned slightly outwards. Pump your arms up and down, without touching the floor, breathing in for 5 counts and out for 5 counts, until you have pumped your arms 100 times. Then lower your feet, bend your knees and relax your upper body onto the floor.

Bridge with single leg

Areas it works
- Abdominals, glutes, hamstrings, balance.

Points to watch
- If you find this tricky, it may help if you raise your leg at an angle of 90 degrees in step 1.
- Keep your upper body relaxed so that your abs and glutes are doing the work.
- Make sure your hips stay level with each other throughout and that you are not sinking into one side.
- Keep the extended leg stretched away from your body.

1 Lie flat on your back with your legs bent and your feet on the floor one hip-width apart. Rest your arms on the floor by your sides. Engage your abdominals and straighten your left leg so that it is in the air at an angle of roughly 45 degrees to the floor.

2 Slowly curl your hips upwards until your knees, hips and shoulders are in a straight line. Keep your hips level. Lower your hips to the floor, then raise them again while keeping your leg in the air. Repeat 5 times on each side.

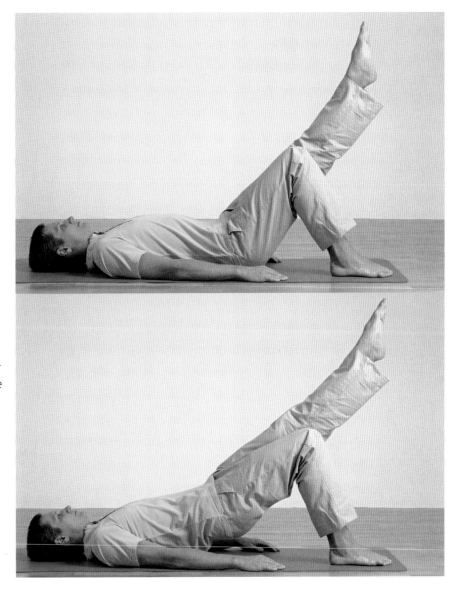

Double leg stretch

Areas it works

- Abdominals, upper torso mobility.

Points to watch

- Keep the upper body and head curved forwards and still throughout the whole exercise.
- Increase the engagement of your abdominals as you progress through the repetitions.

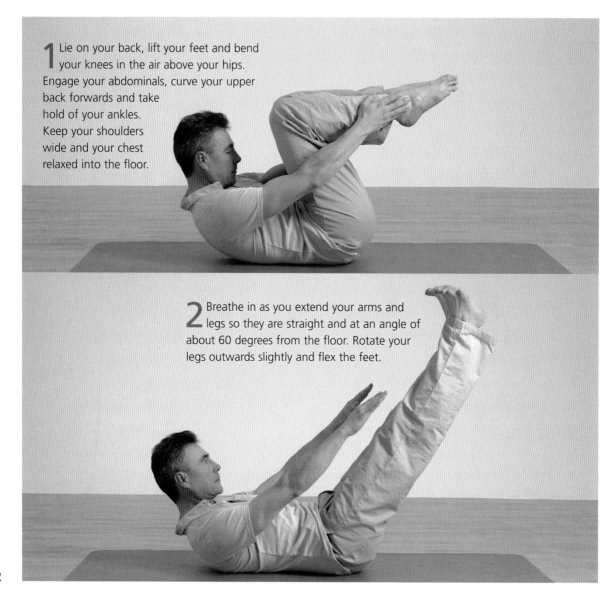

1 Lie on your back, lift your feet and bend your knees in the air above your hips. Engage your abdominals, curve your upper back forwards and take hold of your ankles. Keep your shoulders wide and your chest relaxed into the floor.

2 Breathe in as you extend your arms and legs so they are straight and at an angle of about 60 degrees from the floor. Rotate your legs outwards slightly and flex the feet.

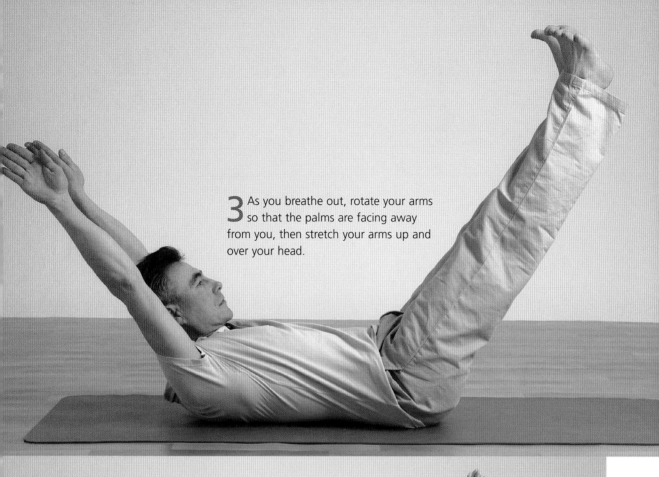

3 As you breathe out, rotate your arms so that the palms are facing away from you, then stretch your arms up and over your head.

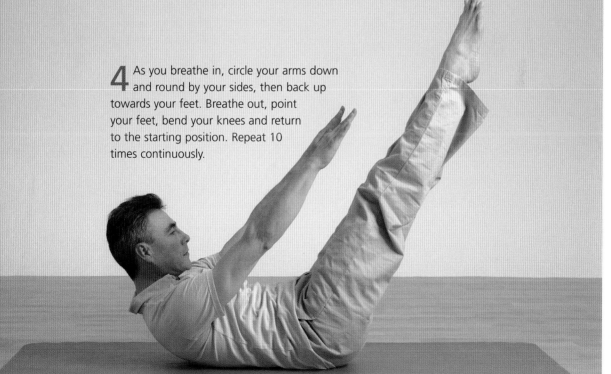

4 As you breathe in, circle your arms down and round by your sides, then back up towards your feet. Breathe out, point your feet, bend your knees and return to the starting position. Repeat 10 times continuously.

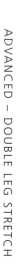

ADVANCED – DOUBLE LEG STRETCH

63

The Saw

Areas it works

- Intercostal muscles, abdominals, obliques, hamstrings.

Points to watch

- Push down into the opposite buttock as you stretch across to keep it anchored to the floor.
- Keep your neck long; don't lead any of the movements with your head.

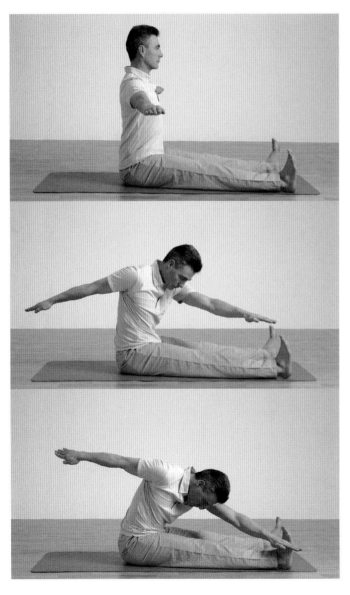

1 Sit up straight on the floor with your legs extended and slightly wider than hip-width apart. Stretch your arms out at your sides at shoulder height. Flex your feet.

2 Breathe in and engage your abdominals, pulling your spine up as tall as you can. As you breathe out, turn to the right from the waist and stretch your left hand over your legs towards the little toe of the right foot.

3 Continue the forwards movement. You should be able to brush past your little toe while still keeping your hips firmly on the floor. Deepen the curve by stretching your head and chest towards your right knee. Breathe in as you draw your body back up to starting position. Then breathe out as you turn to the left and stretch your right hand past your left little toe. Repeat 5 times in each direction.

Side lifts and leg lift

Areas they work
- Outer thighs, obliques, quadratus lumborum.

Points to watch
- Check that your knees, feet and hips are in line with each other. It can help you to keep your balance if you position your legs slightly in front of your pelvis.
- Keep the double lift low, just a few centimetres (2 in) off the floor.

1 Lie on your side with your shoulders, hips, knees and feet aligned and your feet softly pointed forwards. Extend your lower arm straight along the floor under your head, palm down. Rest the fingers of the top hand lightly on the floor in front of you.

2 As you breathe out, engage your abdominals, inner thighs and glutes, then stretch your legs away from your body, lifting them off the floor. At the same time lift your upper body away from your arm.

3 Keeping your lower leg still, lengthen your top leg and raise it as high as you can without moving your hips. Breathing in, lower your top leg again, then point both feet. Lower your upper body and legs to the starting position. Repeat 10 times on each side.

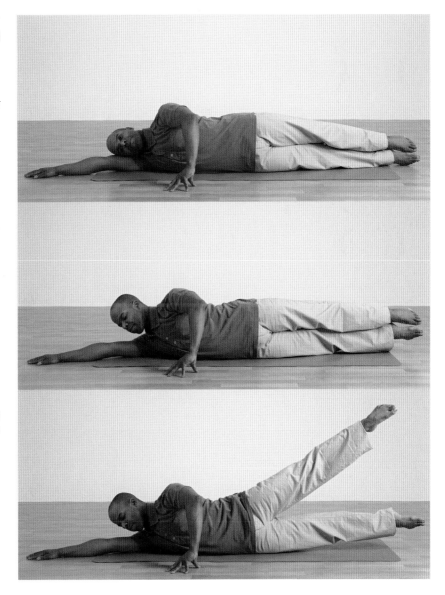

Single leg teaser

Areas it works

• Abdominals, obliques, stamina.

Points to watch

• Lead the lift with your sternum, not your head and neck.
• Use your abdominal muscles to control the raising and lowering movements.
• If you can't manage the Single leg teaser at first, just curve your upper body forwards into a 'C' shape.

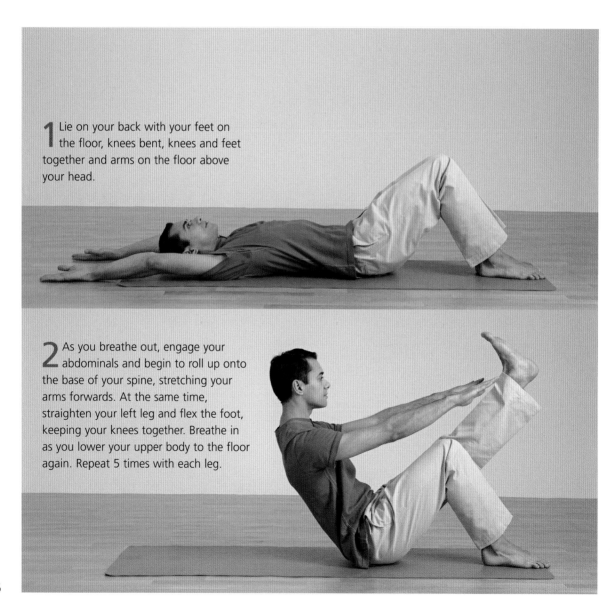

1 Lie on your back with your feet on the floor, knees bent, knees and feet together and arms on the floor above your head.

2 As you breathe out, engage your abdominals and begin to roll up onto the base of your spine, stretching your arms forwards. At the same time, straighten your left leg and flex the foot, keeping your knees together. Breathe in as you lower your upper body to the floor again. Repeat 5 times with each leg.

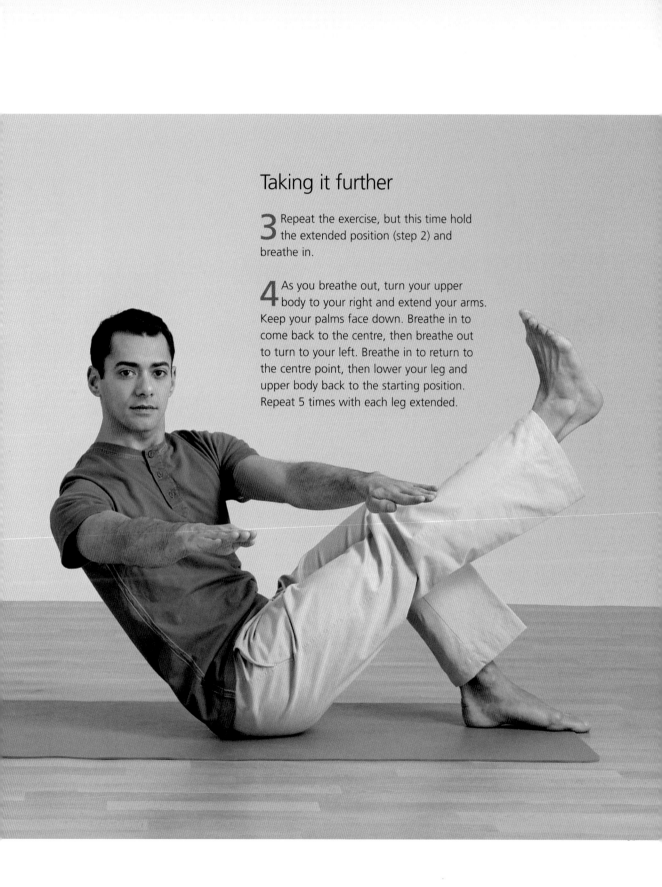

Taking it further

3 Repeat the exercise, but this time hold the extended position (step 2) and breathe in.

4 As you breathe out, turn your upper body to your right and extend your arms. Keep your palms face down. Breathe in to come back to the centre, then breathe out to turn to your left. Breathe in to return to the centre point, then lower your leg and upper body back to the starting position. Repeat 5 times with each leg extended.

Rowing (2)

Areas it works
- Arms, shoulders, hamstrings, back, abdominals.

Points to watch
- Keep your heels firmly on the floor.
- Keep your shoulders down and your neck long.

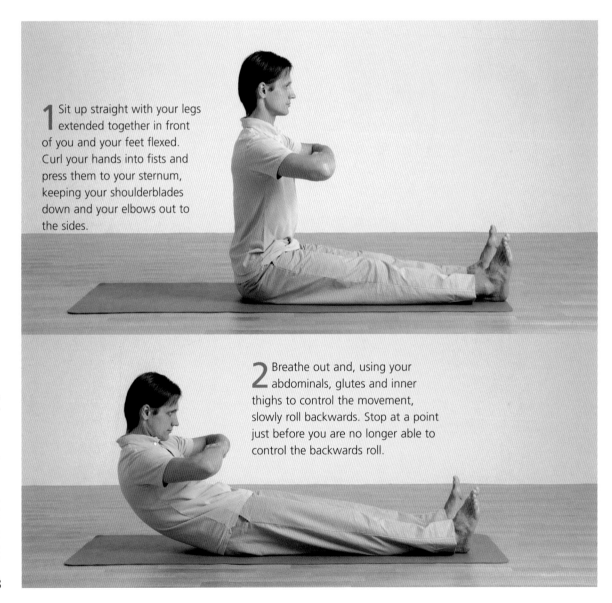

1 Sit up straight with your legs extended together in front of you and your feet flexed. Curl your hands into fists and press them to your sternum, keeping your shoulderblades down and your elbows out to the sides.

2 Breathe out and, using your abdominals, glutes and inner thighs to control the movement, slowly roll backwards. Stop at a point just before you are no longer able to control the backwards roll.

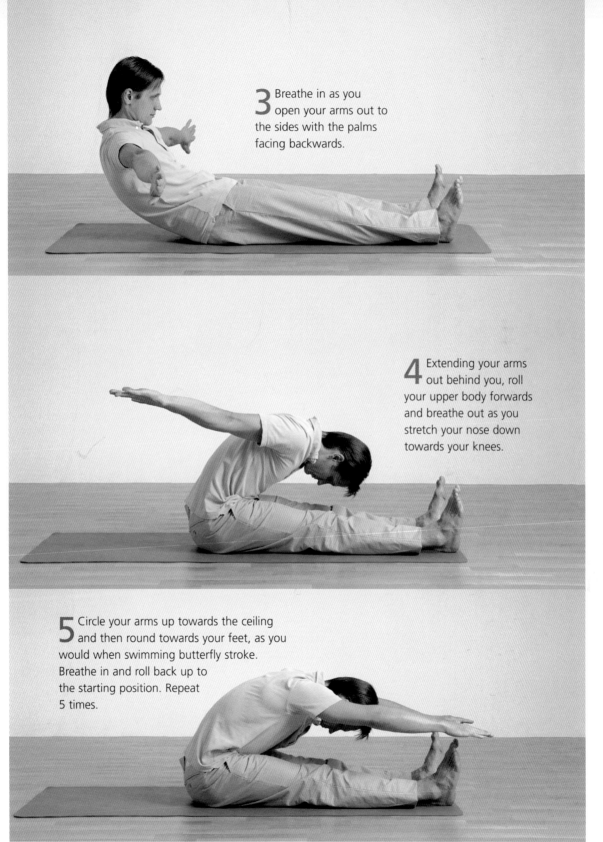

3 Breathe in as you open your arms out to the sides with the palms facing backwards.

4 Extending your arms out behind you, roll your upper body forwards and breathe out as you stretch your nose down towards your knees.

5 Circle your arms up towards the ceiling and then round towards your feet, as you would when swimming butterfly stroke. Breathe in and roll back up to the starting position. Repeat 5 times.

The Twist

Areas it works

- Abdominals, obliques, hips, shoulders and arms, control and balance.

Points to watch

- Keep your hips still and just twist your upper body.
- Don't sink your weight into your arm or shoulder.

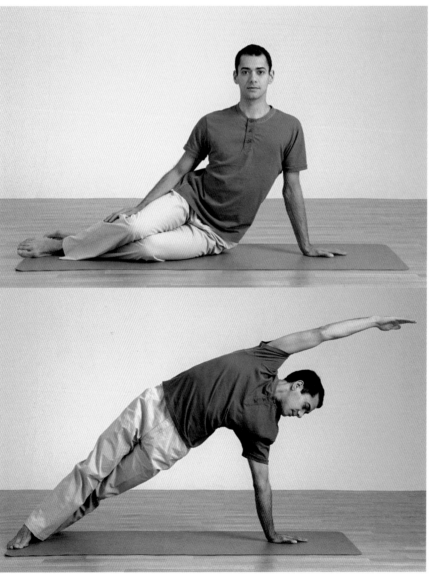

1 Sit on your left hip with your knees bent and together. Place your right foot on the floor just in front of the left. Place your left hand, palm down, on the floor beneath your shoulder, fingers facing away from you, and rest your right hand on your right knee.

2 Breathe in, press down into your left hand, engage your abdominals and push your body up into a straight line. Raise your right arm over your head and turn to look down at your left hand.

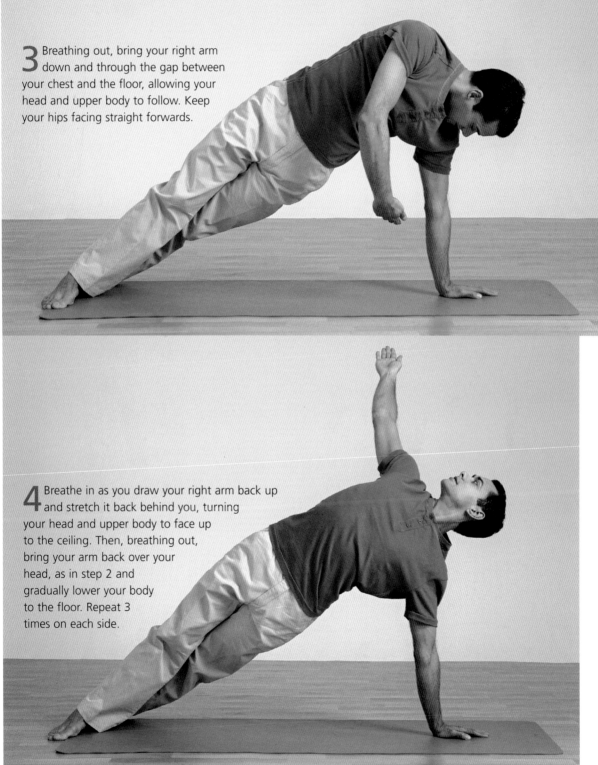

3 Breathing out, bring your right arm down and through the gap between your chest and the floor, allowing your head and upper body to follow. Keep your hips facing straight forwards.

4 Breathe in as you draw your right arm back up and stretch it back behind you, turning your head and upper body to face up to the ceiling. Then, breathing out, bring your arm back over your head, as in step 2 and gradually lower your body to the floor. Repeat 3 times on each side.

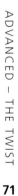

Push-ups

Areas they work

- Arms, shoulders, chest, upper back, abdominals, glutes, hamstrings.

Points to watch

- Your elbows should be virtually pinned to your sides during the push-ups – don't let them stray outwards.
- Keep your spine in a straight line and your neck long.
- Keep your abdominals, glutes and inner thighs firmly engaged throughout the movement.

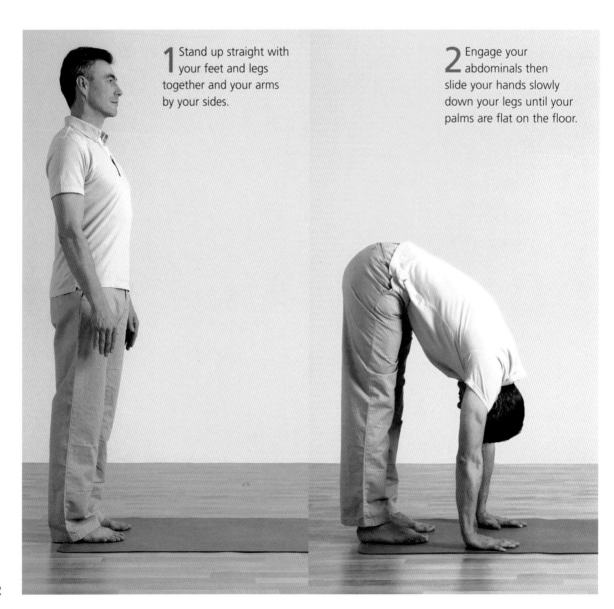

1 Stand up straight with your feet and legs together and your arms by your sides.

2 Engage your abdominals then slide your hands slowly down your legs until your palms are flat on the floor.

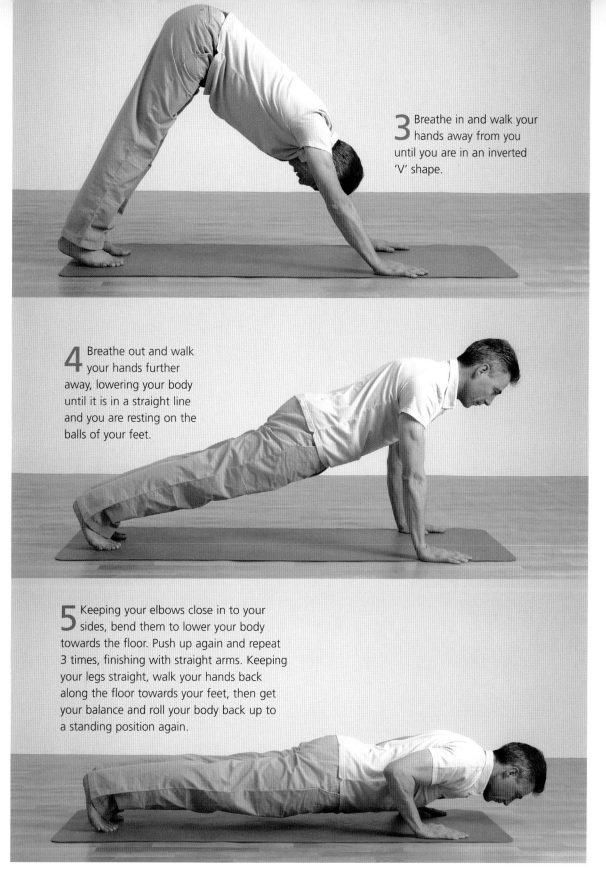

3 Breathe in and walk your hands away from you until you are in an inverted 'V' shape.

4 Breathe out and walk your hands further away, lowering your body until it is in a straight line and you are resting on the balls of your feet.

5 Keeping your elbows close in to your sides, bend them to lower your body towards the floor. Push up again and repeat 3 times, finishing with straight arms. Keeping your legs straight, walk your hands back along the floor towards your feet, then get your balance and roll your body back up to a standing position again.

Chapter 5
Sports specifics

This chapter looks at 13 of the most common sports and offers advice on choosing equipment, using correct techniques and identifying which muscles you should strengthen to improve your game and protect yourself from injury. There's advice on the muscle groups that you need to warm up before you start and stretch out after you finish, along with some specific Pilates exercises you can use. However, it is important for all sports to have good core stability and posture, so you should do regular workouts that strengthen your core muscles. As a basic minimum, include Static abs, Bridging, Glute squeezes, Hamstring curls, The Arrow, Adductors and Hip rolls (1) – all from the Posture workout in Chapter 3 (see pages 30–47) and listed as part of each sport's workout.

Baseball and cricket

These sports have much in common in terms of the muscle groups they use. The most frequent type of injury comes from being hit by the ball, so the most important piece of advice is to wear appropriate protective gear – certainly shin pads, and a mouthguard too if you want to keep your own teeth!

The shoulder is one of the most fragile joints in the human body, with a greater range of movement than any other joint, and bowling can put a lot of strain on it because of the internal rotation required while the arm is extended at an angle. It is a ball and socket joint where three bones – the humerus of the upper arm, the scapula (shoulderblade) and clavicle (collarbone) – are held together by four tendons known as the rotator cuff. Keeping the surrounding muscle groups balanced is important so that uneven pressure isn't placed on the rotator cuff, which could cause it to become inflamed, or could even lead to dislocation of the humerus.

Do you bowl front on, with your head, chest and feet facing forwards? Or side on, with your back foot parallel to the crease and your upper body rotated? The more twisting there is in your bowling action, the more strain you are putting on the lumbar spine, hips and knees, so the stronger the muscles in those areas need to be to be able to withstand the pressure.

Knee problems can also affect fielders, who have the additional challenge that they can be standing around for long periods and are then required to make sudden movements. It's important to keep active on the field so that the muscles stay warmed up and you are ready to spring for that spectacular catch when it comes your way.

The workout

- Static abs *(see page 31)*
- Bridging *(see page 32)*
- Glute squeezes *(see page 35)*
- Hamstring curls *(see page 36)*
- The Arrow *(see page 38)*
- Adductors *(see page 39)*
- Hip rolls (1) *(see page 42)*
- Arm and elbow circles *(see pages 76–77)*
- Rowing (1) *(see pages 58–59)*
- Arm weights *(see page 78)*
- The Saw *(see page 64)*
- Swimming *(see page 55)*
- Sitting lats *(see page 45)*
- Arm openings *(see page 46)*
- Twisting with a pole *(see page 85)*

Arm circles

This exercise will help to loosen up your shoulders before a game or match in any sport that puts stress on the shoulder joint. It's also good for loosening tense shoulders during a stressful day at the office.

Contraindications
• If you have any kind of impingement of the shoulder joint, keep the movement very small and contained. Stop *before* it hurts.

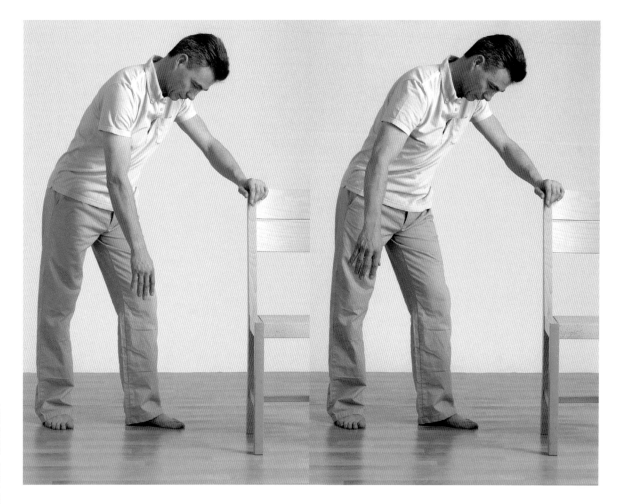

1 Stand with your left hand on the back of a chair, and your left leg bent, roughly 30 cm (1 ft) in front of the right leg. Lean forwards and let your right arm hang down loosely from the shoulder.

2 Circle your right arm a few times clockwise and then anticlockwise. Repeat with the left arm.

Elbow circles

If you have mild to moderately stiff shoulders, try this exercise to increase the ease of movement. If you find it difficult to touch your fingertips to your shoulder joints, hold them slightly higher rather than trying to force them down.

Contraindications

• As with Arm circles, keep the movement small if you have shoulder impingement.
• Don't force the elbow joint to bend if you find this difficult.
• Avoid hunching the shoulders to get into the starting position.

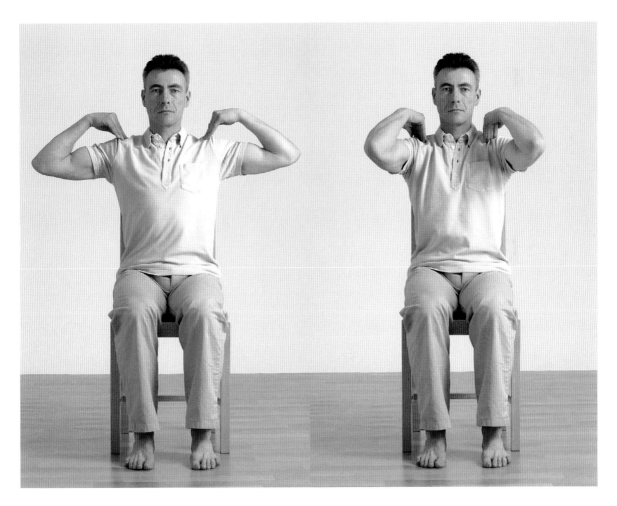

1 Sit on a chair with your back straight, bend your elbows out to the sides in line with your shoulders and place your fingertips on top of your shoulder joints.

2 Draw circles in the air with your elbows, first forwards and then backwards. Don't try to make the circles too big – the shoulder joint shouldn't click at all. Keep your shoulders back and avoid hunching forwards while making the circles.

Arm weights

For these exercises, you will need hand weights of not more than 3 kg (6½ lb) each. If you don't have any, you could substitute a can of soup or beans from the storecupboard.

Contraindications

• Don't try this if you have repetitive strain injury or any kind of wrist problem, tennis elbow or any other kind of elbow problem. Be careful that your elbows don't 'snap' as you straighten.

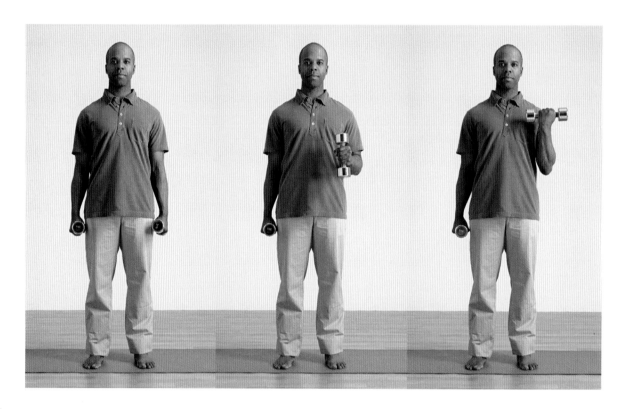

1 Stand with your back straight and your feet on the floor hip-width apart. Let your arms hang down straight by your sides. Hold the weights with your palms facing in towards your thighs.

2 Engage your abdominals and bend your left elbow until your arm is at a right angle.

3 Rotate your forearm so your palm is facing upwards, and continue the movement towards your left shoulder. Lower your left arm as you raise the right weight towards your right shoulder, using the same method. Alternate arms and keep your shoulders relaxed throughout. Try to make the movements smooth and flowing. Repeat 10 times with each arm.

Deltoids

These movements are very simple and you should be able to do them easily, but don't be tempted to use heavier weights. Increase the number of repetitions if you want more of a challenge.

Contraindications
• Avoid this if you suffer shoulder impingement.
• Keep your wrists in a straight line when holding the weights; don't let them bend forwards.

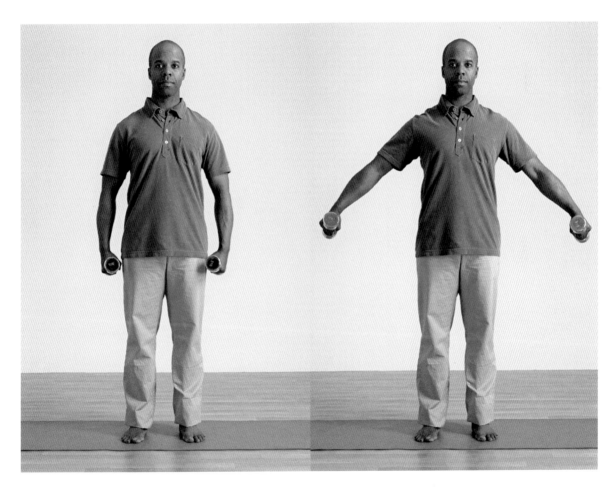

1 Stand up straight with your back about 30 cm (1 ft) in front of a wall, and with your feet hip-width apart. Slightly bend your knees. Let your arms hang down by your sides with slightly bent elbows and hold the hand weights with your palms facing in towards your thighs.

2 Engage your abdominals, pull down your shoulder-blades and slowly raise your arms out to the sides until they are midway to your shoulders. Avoid letting your shoulders lift up. Lower your arms to your sides again and repeat 10 times.

Cycling

In chapter 2 I explained how the repetitive movements you make when you sit with a bad posture are a sure-fire way to cause injury. If you sit with bad posture on a bike and perform strenuous pedalling movements for extended periods of time, you're almost certainly heading for a fall.

The first step to good cycling technique is choosing the right bike. When you stand over a bike, there should be a clearance of 2–8 cm (¾–3 in) between your crotch and the bar. When sitting on the seat with your feet on the ground, your knees should be slightly bent. When you hold the handlebars and put your feet on the pedals, 40 per cent of your weight should be distributed forwards over the front wheel and 60 per cent over the back wheel. (I know this is tricky to measure, but you should be able to judge from the feel.)

Choose a seat that feels comfortable to you. Recumbent bikes with laid-back seating provide good back support. A suspension seat is best for recreational rather than racing cycling, and bikes with shock absorbers will be much easier on your bones and joints.

When sitting on the bike, keep your spine in a naturally straight line and think of lengthening through your neck and upper spine. Don't hunch over the bars with your head dropped and your chin sticking out or you'll soon get back, shoulder and neck strain, and could become a candidate for kyphosis (see page 24).

As you pedal, your knees should remain in line with the middle of your foot and not drift in or out or you'll be putting strain on the knee ligaments. The higher the seat, the less your knees will have to bend, so the less stress you will put on them. If you have existing hip, knee, ankle or foot problems, such as bowed legs, knock knees or flat feet, it may be difficult for you to achieve a good cycling technique.

Finally, watch the surfaces you cycle on. Rocky, bumpy tracks will impact on your joints and may also cause you to fall off. Stand on the pedals before hitting a bump and your entire body will act as a shock absorber.

The workout

- **Static abs** *(see page 31)*
- **Bridging** *(see page 32)*
- **Glute squeezes** *(see page 35)*
- **Hamstring curls** *(see page 36)*
- **The Arrow** *(see page 38)*
- **Adductors** *(see page 39)*
- **Hip rolls (1)** *(see page 42)*
- **Pillow squeezes** *(see page 81)*
- **Wrist strengthener** *(see page 95)*
- **Upper torso release** *(see pages 82–83)*
- **Lying pecs** *(see page 95)*
- **Chest opening exercise** *(see page 91)*
- **Swimming** *(see page 55)*
- **Push-ups** *(see pages 72–73)*
- **Quad stretches** *(see pages 122–23)*
- **Calf stretches** *(see pages 128–29)*

Pillow squeezes

Leaning forwards over the handlebars can lead to shoulder tension, but this exercise helps to counteract it by pulling the shoulderblades away from the spine and strengthening the serratus anterior muscles.

Contraindications

- Don't tense in the neck as you squeeze. If you feel tension, turn your head slightly towards the side you are squeezing.
- Don't arch your lower back – keep it straight but soft throughout the exercise.

1 Sit up straight on a stool with your feet flat on the floor one hip-width apart. Fold a pillow in half and place it under your right arm, with your elbow bent at right angles, so that you are holding it between your elbow and your ribs. Engage your abdominals and squeeze the pillow. Hold for 5 seconds then relax. You should feel your shoulderblade moving. Repeat 10 times on each side.

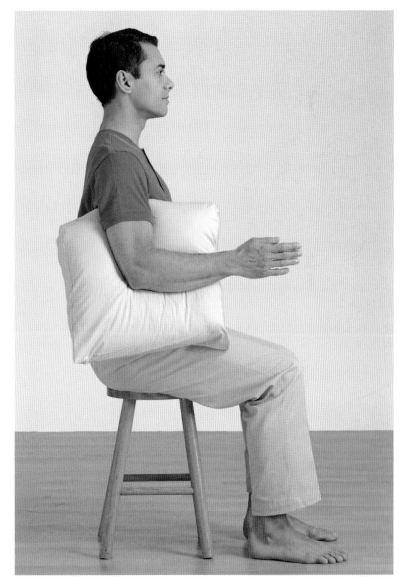

Upper torso release

This is another exercise that is good for freeing tight shoulderblades and relieving upper back tension. You should be able to feel the side-to-side movement releasing the muscles between your shoulderblades.

Contraindications

- Don't try this if you have serious shoulder problems. Reduce the range of movement if your shoulder clicks.
- If you have neck problems, lie with a small pillow or a paperback book under your head.

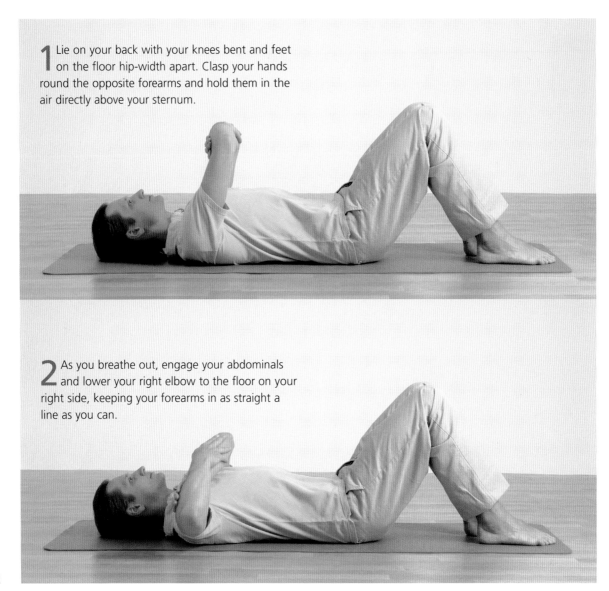

1 Lie on your back with your knees bent and feet on the floor hip-width apart. Clasp your hands round the opposite forearms and hold them in the air directly above your sternum.

2 As you breathe out, engage your abdominals and lower your right elbow to the floor on your right side, keeping your forearms in as straight a line as you can.

3 Breathe in to return to the centre, then breathe out to lower your left elbow to the floor on your left side.

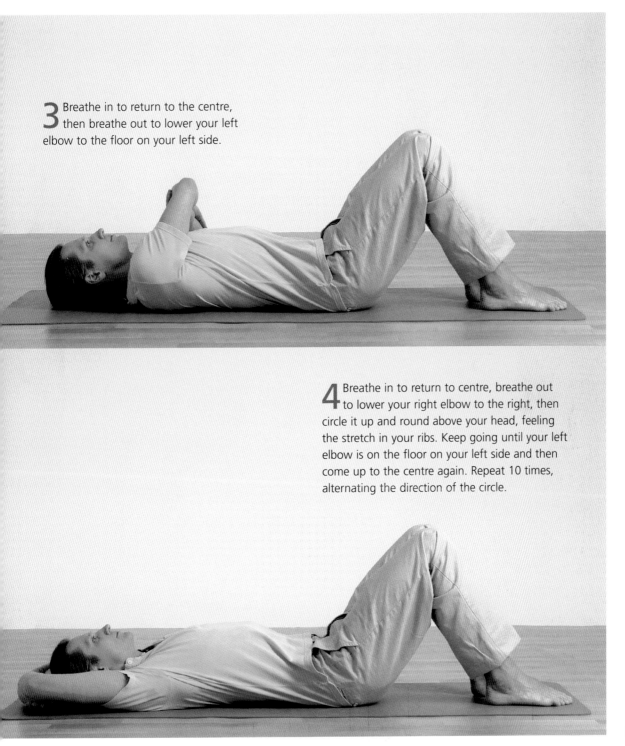

4 Breathe in to return to centre, breathe out to lower your right elbow to the right, then circle it up and round above your head, feeling the stretch in your ribs. Keep going until your left elbow is on the floor on your left side and then come up to the centre again. Repeat 10 times, alternating the direction of the circle.

Football

As you can tell from the number of seasoned professional footballers who have to sit out a match or a season, injuries can occur to the best players at the top of their game. That means they are even more common for Saturday morning amateurs, who may not have had any exercise during the week, and those men launch into the new season each autumn after lazing on a sunbed all summer instead of training. Fitness and muscle strength are crucial for a sport in which you have to run at full speed while kicking a ball, swerve to avoid a tackle, jump high in the air, turn suddenly to face the goal and then kick with maximum power.

The most common football injuries occur to the groin, knees and lower legs. Knees can suffer progressive wear and tear as the cartilage (or meniscus) covering the surface of the bones gets torn either partially or fully and little bits of 'gravel' end up floating inside the joint cavity. Knee ligament damage can occur when the foot is fixed to the ground by the boot studs and the body twists sideways over it. Accidentally standing on another player's foot, or their standing on yours, can cause ankle and knee problems for both of you.

Make sure you kick the ball with the correct part of your foot, which is towards the front of the instep. Repeatedly kicking with the top or inside of the foot will irritate the ankle, while kicking with the toes can break your toes. You need strength and flexibility in the feet and the ankles to prevent injury when turning while running, or landing awkwardly after a jump – as can occur when you leap upwards to try and head that corner kick into the goal and collide with a team mate in mid-air.

The workout

- Static abs *(see page 31)*
- Bridging *(see page 32)*
- Glute squeezes *(see page 35)*
- Hamstring curls *(see page 36)*
- The Arrow *(see page 38)*
- Adductors *(see page 39)*
- Hip rolls (1) *(see page 42)*
- Swimming *(see page 55)*
- Rolling like a ball *(see page 53)*
- The Hundred *(see page 49 and page 60)*
- Criss-cross *(see page 52)*
- Double leg stretch *(see pages 62–63)*
- Twisting with a pole *(see page 85)* followed by quadratus lumborum stretch *(see pages 126–27)*
- Isometric neck exercises *(see pages 86–87)* followed by Neck stretch *(see pages 134–35)*
- Ankle strengthener *(see page 107)*
- Tensor fascia lata stretch *(see pages 118–19)*
- Hamstring and Quad stretches *(see pages 120–23)*

Twisting with a pole

You'll need a pole that's approximately 1 metre (3 ft) long – a broom handle would do. This exercise helps to develop the rotational flexibility of your spine.

Contraindications
• Don't try this if you have disc compression in your lumbar spine or any other kind of lower back problems.

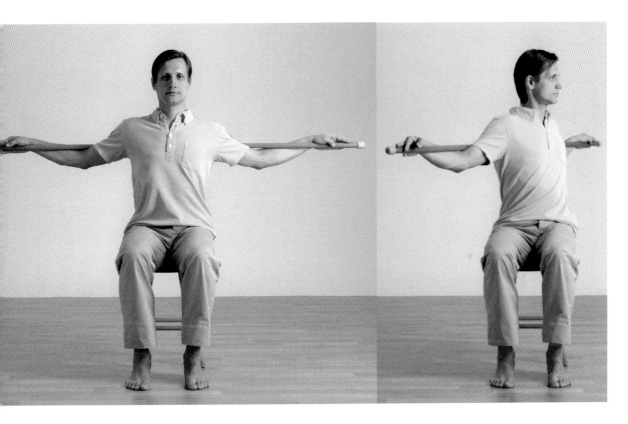

1 Sit up straight on a chair with your feet on the floor positioned hip-width apart. Place the pole across your back roughly at the base of the shoulderblades and hold it in position with your lower arms over it and your elbows bent underneath. Your forearms should be parallel to the floor and your palms face down.

2 As you breathe out, engage your abdominals and turn your upper body to the left, keeping your hips still and your spine long – imagine your upper body twisting around your spine. Breathe in to return to the centre. Breathe out to twist round to the right. Repeat 5 times in each direction.

Isometric neck exercises

Most football training focuses on the legs, abdominals and aerobic fitness. Few footballers think about the neck muscles, but these need to be strong for heading the ball, so include the following simple exercises in your workout at least once a week.

Contraindications

• There are no real contraindications to this exercise, but make sure you sit with correct posture. The pressure between head and hand shouldn't be very strong.

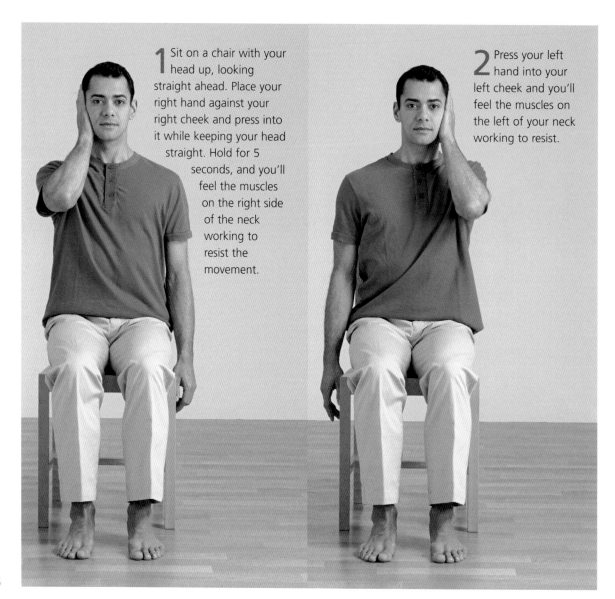

1 Sit on a chair with your head up, looking straight ahead. Place your right hand against your right cheek and press into it while keeping your head straight. Hold for 5 seconds, and you'll feel the muscles on the right side of the neck working to resist the movement.

2 Press your left hand into your left cheek and you'll feel the muscles on the left of your neck working to resist.

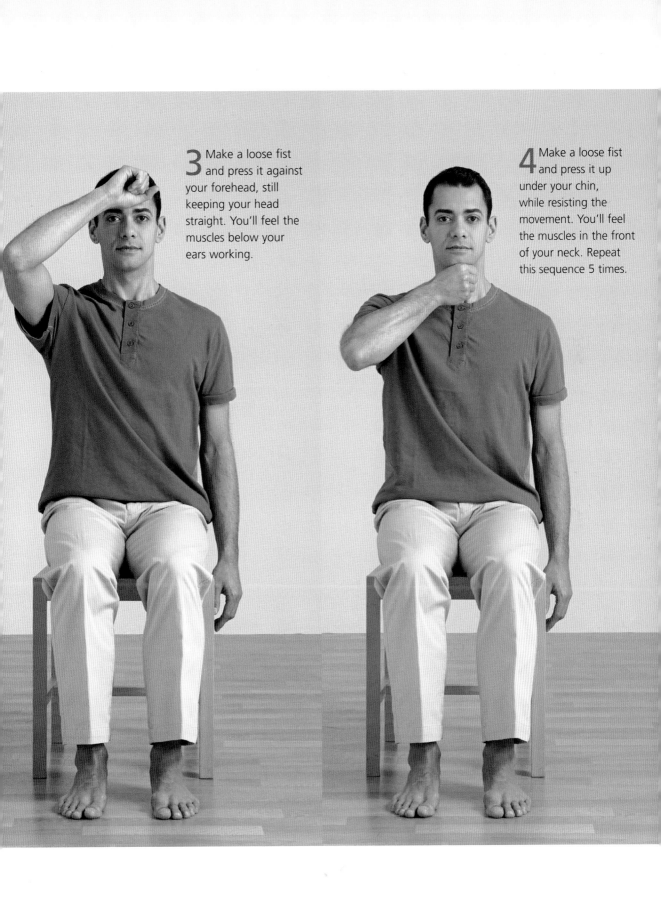

3 Make a loose fist and press it against your forehead, still keeping your head straight. You'll feel the muscles below your ears working.

4 Make a loose fist and press it up under your chin, while resisting the movement. You'll feel the muscles in the front of your neck. Repeat this sequence 5 times.

Golf

Professional lessons to improve your golf swing could be one of the best investments you ever make. A poor golf swing can cause back, neck and shoulder injuries – as well as seriously damaging your game. During the swing, your lumbar spine bends to one side, rotates, compresses and moves backwards and forwards. The leading shoulder goes through an extreme range of motion, while the neck has to stay fairly still or you'll take your eyes off the ball and probably miss it.

You may not think of golf as a particularly energetic game, but a good warm-up is essential to stretch out the muscles or you risk nasty tears and spinal injuries. Putting with good posture is a recommended warm-up technique, and if you go to a driving range, start with short swings before building up to full ones.

Vibration is transmitted through your wrist and forearm when you strike the ball, and this will be exacerbated if you're gripping too hard or at a peculiar angle. Get a pro to check your grip.

Finally, lifting and carrying heavy golf bags, and regularly bending over to pick up balls can be disastrous for a weak lower back. Follow the rules for correct lifting: bend your knees so that you're level with the object and it's right in front of you, then keep your spine straight as you straighten your legs to stand up.

The workout

- **Static abs** (see page 31)
- **Bridging** (see page 32)
- **Glute squeezes** (see page 35)
- **Hamstring curls** (see page 36)
- **The Arrow** (see page 38)
- **Adductors** (see page 39)
- **Hip rolls (1)** (see page 42)
- **Rowing (1)** (see pages 58–59)
- **Swimming** (see page 55)
- **Push-ups** (see pages 72–73)
- **Arm weights** (see page 78)
- **The Saw** (see page 64)
- **Twisting with a pole** (see page 85)
- **Balance tests** (see page 89)
- **Chest opening exercise** (see page 90)
- **Chest opening with circle exercise** (see page 91)

Balance tests

You'll need strong core stability to perform this perfectly. If you find it easier to stand on one leg than the other, do extra repetitions on the weaker leg.

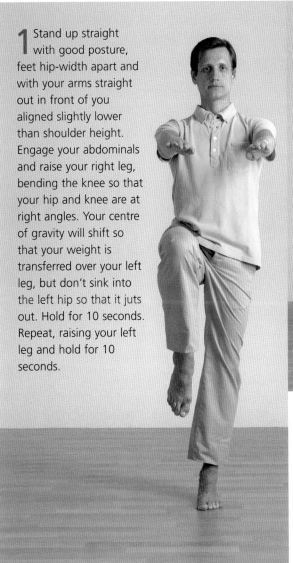

1 Stand up straight with good posture, feet hip-width apart and with your arms straight out in front of you aligned slightly lower than shoulder height. Engage your abdominals and raise your right leg, bending the knee so that your hip and knee are at right angles. Your centre of gravity will shift so that your weight is transferred over your left leg, but don't sink into the left hip so that it juts out. Hold for 10 seconds. Repeat, raising your left leg and hold for 10 seconds.

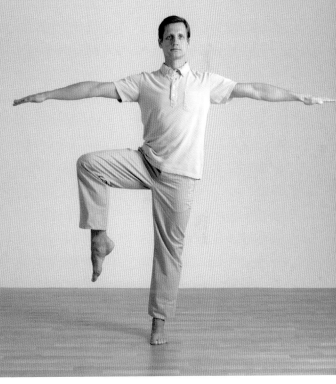

2 Hold your arms out to your sides at shoulder height. Engage your abdominals and raise your right leg out to the side so that your hip and knee are at right angles and your thigh is parallel to your right arm. Hold for 10 seconds. Repeat on your left leg. Repeat the whole sequence 5 times.

GOLF

89

Chest opening exercise

This is beneficial for any sport that involves a forward swing of the shoulder, as it reverses the movement and releases tightness in the chest and shoulders.

Contraindications

• Avoid this if you suffer from lumbar spine weakness or from a shoulder impingement. Don't feel you have to lower your hand all the way back to the floor. Stop at any point if it feels uncomfortable.

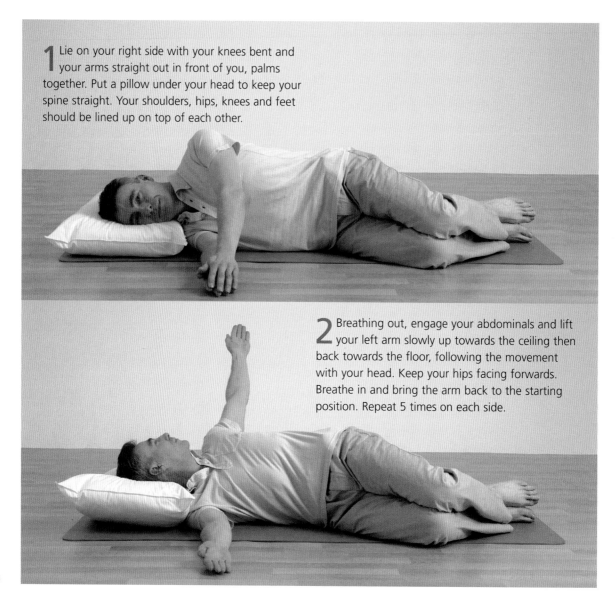

1 Lie on your right side with your knees bent and your arms straight out in front of you, palms together. Put a pillow under your head to keep your spine straight. Your shoulders, hips, knees and feet should be lined up on top of each other.

2 Breathing out, engage your abdominals and lift your left arm slowly up towards the ceiling then back towards the floor, following the movement with your head. Keep your hips facing forwards. Breathe in and bring the arm back to the starting position. Repeat 5 times on each side.

Chest opening exercise with circle

This takes the Chest opening exercise a stage further. You should be able to feel a good stretch in your ribs and shoulders and after a few weeks of practice you will probably find that your shoulder mobility has much increased.

Contraindications
• As for Chest opening exercise.

1 Lie on your right side with your knees bent and your arms straight out on the floor in front of you and your palms together.

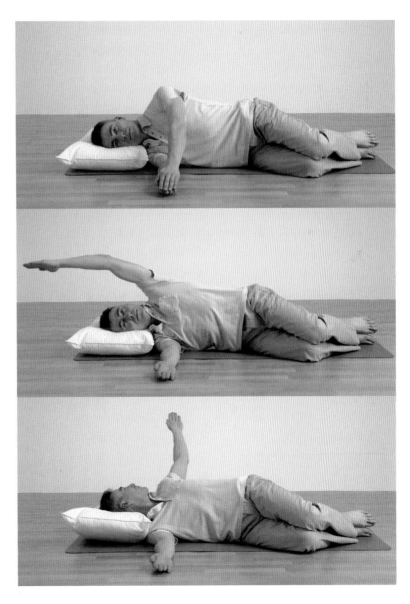

2 Breathe in, and as you breathe out begin to draw your upper arm up above your head. Continue circling your arm over your face and round above the top of your head.

3 Pause to breathe in, then continue the movement behind you as far as you can go before bringing your arm back over your body to the starting position. Repeat the movement 5 times, then turn onto your left side and do the whole exercise lying on your left side and moving your right arm.

Gym

If you are keen to spend time in the gym getting fit, make sure that a gym instructor explains how to use each piece of equipment and change the settings to suit your physique, and then supervises you until you know what you are doing. It's also essential that you do a warm-up of about 15 minutes (see right) before you begin your workout.

The key thing to remember is that you should only use the set of muscles you are targeting for each particular exercise, and you shouldn't feel strain elsewhere. If veins or tendons are standing out on your neck or you feel any tension in your back, then you are performing the exercise incorrectly. Men can be so competitive that you see them working out with weights that they can hardly lift, and their eyes are virtually popping out of their heads. This doesn't prove that they're strong. More repetitions with manageable weights will give much better results.

Engage your abdominals when using any gym equipment to help keep your posture correct and protect your back from strain.

Here's the low-down on the correct and incorrect ways of using some of the more common pieces of gym equipment.

Free weights
Use these weights to perform Bicep curls: pick a weight that feels moderately heavy, hold a weight in each hand and raise one arm at a time with your palm facing up and your elbows held close to your body. Make sure you're not leaning backwards or using your shoulders in the lift.

Pectoral press machine
Sit on the machine with good posture and with your elbows and forearms against the pads. Push the pads together until they touch in front of your chest. Keep your spine straight and don't let your head or shoulders tilt forwards.

Treadmill
Use proper running technique, placing your heel down first then rolling through your foot and pushing off with your toes. Don't lean forwards, which could strain your calf muscles. Keep your shoulders relaxed and down, and your eye line straight forwards.

Rowing machine
Keep your spine straight – don't lean your upper body back or bend your neck forwards. Pull the bar directly to your chest, not any higher or lower. Keep your knees in line with your feet, rather than letting them open outwards as you come forwards.

A warm-up for gym work

- Static abs *(see page 31)*
- Hamstring curls *(see page 36)*
- Sitting lats *(see page 45)*
- Adductors *(see page 39)*
- Finally, loosen up any areas that feel tight with the appropriate stretches from Chapter 6 *(see pages 116–135).*

Bench press

In the gym, this is performed lying on a bench and lifting dumbbells but it can be done at home with hand weights.

Contraindications
• Avoid this if you have elbow, wrist or shoulder problems.

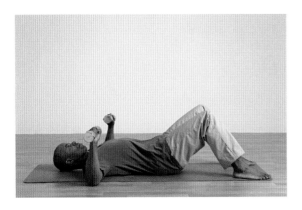

1 Lie on your back with your knees bent and feet flat on the floor. Rest your elbows on the floor at your sides and hold some weights with an overhand grip, palms forward.

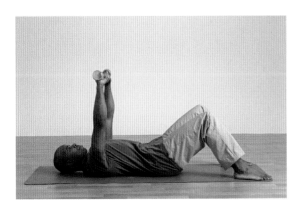

2 Breathe out and engage your abdominals, keeping your shoulders down as you push the weights up until your arms are straight. Keep your back in contact with the floor at all times, without forcing your lower back down or letting it arch. Breathe in to return to the starting position. Repeat 10 times.

Tricep dips

In a gym, you stand up in the Tricep dip equipment. This is a substitute you can try at home using a chair or the edge of a bench.

Contraindications
• Avoid this if you have wrist, elbow or shoulder problems.

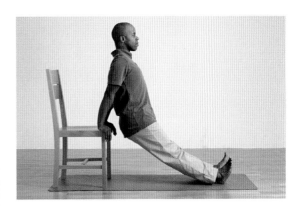

1 Sit on a chair, with your hands holding the edge on either side of your hips. Stretch your legs out on the floor in front of you. Slide your hips off the seat.

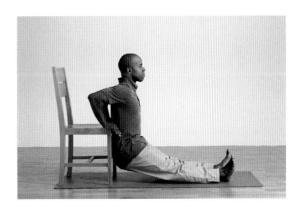

2 Bend your elbows and lower your pelvis, keeping your hips close to the chair. Don't let your wrists bend backwards. Straighten your arms to return to the starting position. Repeat 5 times.

Hockey

A lot of hockey injuries to the body are caused by being hit by the ball or whacked with a hockey stick. Shin pads are a good idea, and so is keeping your eye on the ball, especially when it's up in the air and coming your way.

Like footballers, hockey players need to have strong leg muscles in order to accelerate, swerve and turn suddenly, and you need flexibility in your hip muscles as well as good core stability. You are prone to knee ligament and cartilage problems, ankle and groin sprains, so it's important to keep the leg muscle groups strong and balanced.

On top of this, you have to stoop slightly to dribble the ball along the pitch and pass it to other players. This can strain the back muscles over time if you don't have very good core stability. After a match, exercises such as The Cobra, The Arrow and Swimming can help to counteract the effects of leaning forwards on the pitch. Make no mistake: hockey requires a high degree of fitness, both strength and aerobic, and a good coach should test his team regularly to make sure they are up to the challenges.

The workout

- Static abs *(see page 31)*
- Bridging *(see page 32)*
- Glute squeezes *(see page 35)*
- Hamstring curls *(see page 36)*
- The Arrow *(see page 38)*
- Adductors *(see page 39)*
- Hip rolls (1) *(see page 42)*
- The Cobra *(see page 37)*
- Swimming *(see page 55)*
- Arm weights *(see page 78)*
- Lying pecs *(see page 95)*
- Wrist strengthener *(see page 95)*
- Hamstring and Quad stretches *(see pages 120–23)*

Lying pecs

Wrist strengthener

This exercise opens the chest and could counteract any forwards curvature of the upper back. You'll need two hand-held weights of not more than 3 kg (6½ lb) each.

You'll need a length of dowelling that has a weight suspended on a string from its centre.

Contraindications
• Avoid this if you have weak wrists or elbows.

Contraindications
• Don't do this if you can't hold your arms straight out due to a neck or upper back problem.

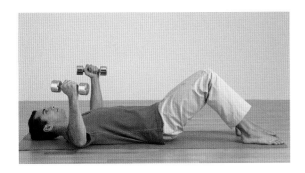

1 Lie on your back with your knees bent and your feet flat on the floor. Holding a weight in each hand, palms facing inwards, curve your arms above your chest, keeping your elbows wide and your shoulders relaxed.

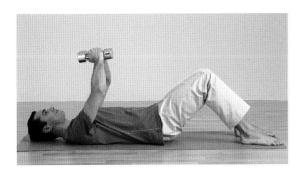

2 Breathing out, engage your abdominals and open your elbows out to touch the floor, maintaining a curve shape in your arms. Breathe in to bring your arms back to centre. Repeat 5 times then do another 5 repetitions with the breathing pattern reversed.

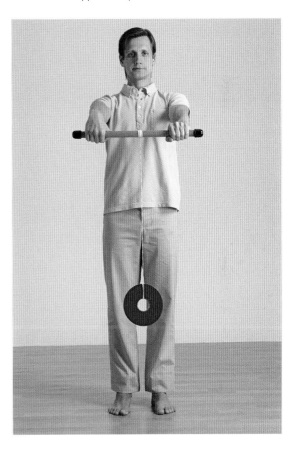

Hold the dowelling in front of you slightly below shoulder level. Your palms should face down. Roll the dowelling, alternating your hands, to raise the weight up. When the weight reaches the level of the dowelling, unroll the string again and repeat 5 times.

Rugby

Scrums can cause some horrible injuries if they collapse badly; in the most extreme cases, players can break their necks. More common are broken collarbones or dislocated shoulders when you fall at an awkward angle onto your outstretched hand and the impact is transmitted up the arm. It's important to learn how to fall on your shoulder and roll to dissipate the impact.

Rugby players should keep up their training out of season and between matches to maintain match fitness. As the game is played in cold, wintry weather, it's doubly important to warm up your muscles before a match.

Hamstring injuries are extremely common in sports such as rugby, when you have to accelerate suddenly from stationary to full sprint in a few seconds. Exercises and stretches that lengthen the hamstrings and strengthen the hip rotator muscles will help to protect you. Sudden changes in direction can put pressure on the knees, especially if your spikes are fixed in the ground while your body weight goes the other way, and calf and ankle injuries can also be caused in this fashion. Groin injuries are usually caused by the quads overworking while the hamstrings and inner thighs aren't working enough, so it's important to do plenty of work on the hamstrings, adductors and calves.

The workout

- **Static abs** *(see page 31)*
- **Bridging** *(see page 32)*
- **Glute squeezes** *(see page 35)*
- **Hamstring curls** *(see page 36)*
- **The Arrow** *(see page 38)*
- **Adductors** *(see page 39)*
- **Hip rolls (1)** *(see page 42)*
- **The Cobra** *(see page 37)*
- **The Cat** *(see page 109)*
- **Hamstring stretches** *(see pages 120–21)*
- **Spine twist** *(see pages 98–99)*
- **Obliques** *(see page 97)*
- **Ankle strengthener** *(see page 107)*
- **Quadratus lumborum stretch** *(see pages 126–27)*

Obliques

Strengthening the oblique muscles helps your body to rotate and bend to the sides. It can also help to define your waist and get rid of love handles!

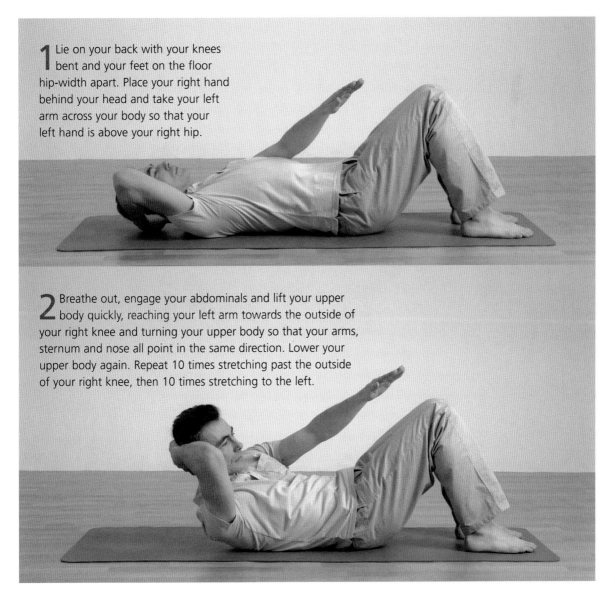

1 Lie on your back with your knees bent and your feet on the floor hip-width apart. Place your right hand behind your head and take your left arm across your body so that your left hand is above your right hip.

2 Breathe out, engage your abdominals and lift your upper body quickly, reaching your left arm towards the outside of your right knee and turning your upper body so that your arms, sternum and nose all point in the same direction. Lower your upper body again. Repeat 10 times stretching past the outside of your right knee, then 10 times stretching to the left.

Spine twist

Rugby players can become very bulky and inflexible round the middle, so any exercises that focus on flexibility will be helpful. Just go as far as you can with this one and you should loosen up over time.

Contraindications

• Avoid the Spin twist exercise if you are prone to pain in your lumbar spine, or if you are unable to hold your hands out to the sides without feeling tension in your shoulders.

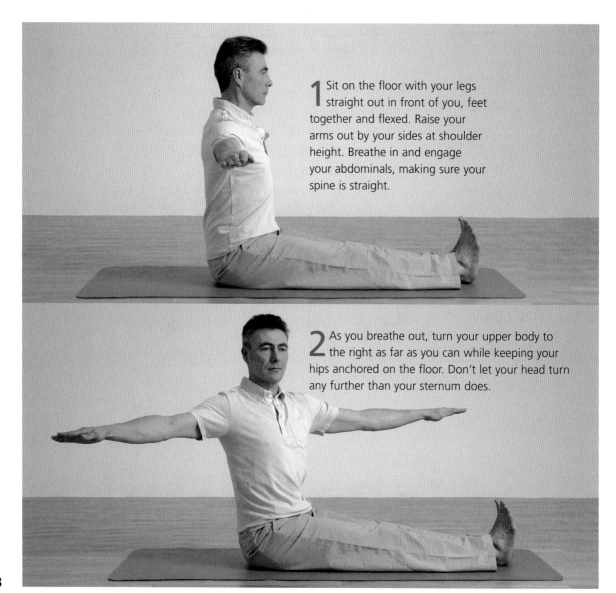

1 Sit on the floor with your legs straight out in front of you, feet together and flexed. Raise your arms out by your sides at shoulder height. Breathe in and engage your abdominals, making sure your spine is straight.

2 As you breathe out, turn your upper body to the right as far as you can while keeping your hips anchored on the floor. Don't let your head turn any further than your sternum does.

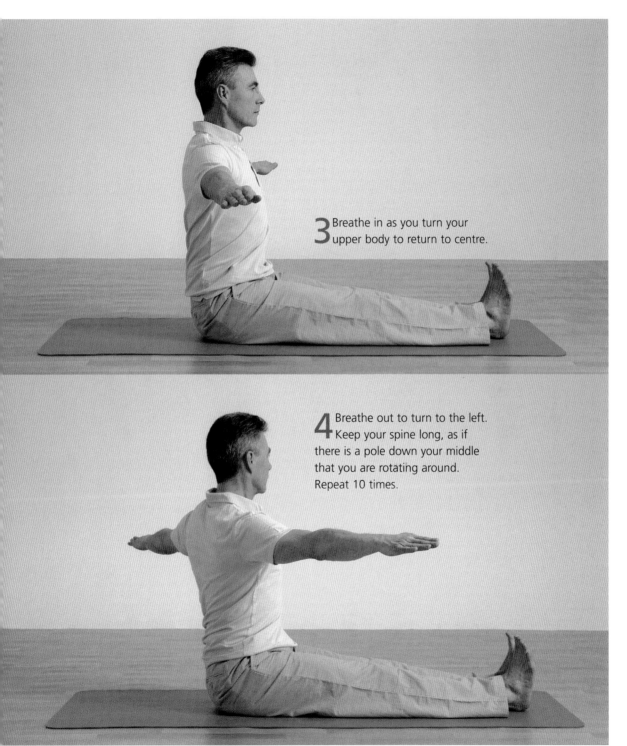

3 Breathe in as you turn your upper body to return to centre.

4 Breathe out to turn to the left. Keep your spine long, as if there is a pole down your middle that you are rotating around. Repeat 10 times.

Running

Running is probably the most popular form of exercise, and it's a great heart and lung workout. The only equipment you need is a good pair of running shoes that fit well and feel comfortable, supporting your foot through its range of movement and offering enough flexibility to allow you to roll through from heel to toe. Normal trainers won't do because they don't have flexible-enough soles. It's worth going to a specialist running shoe retailer to get advice on the best type of shoe for your feet; for example, if you have a tendency to roll your feet in or out, the specialist can recommend particular shoes or insoles to compensate for this.

The ideal running surface is flat and even with a bit of give, and without any camber or obstacles in the way. Running tracks are best, but if you run in the local park or on city streets, beware of broken paving stones, rocks and stray dogs that could cause nasty injuries if you hit them at speed.

Always warm up thoroughly to increase blood flow and oxygen supply to the muscles and loosen up joints. Concentrate on stretching the tensor fascia lata, hamstrings, quads and lower back, all of which have to act as shock absorbers from the impact of your feet hitting the ground.

Running can highlight existing postural problems, such as uneven leg lengths, so any aches or pains you incur should be investigated. If you are consistently aching after your run, try getting specialist advice to correct your running technique.

The workout

- Static abs *(see page 31)*
- Bridging *(see page 32)*
- Glute squeezes *(see page 35)*
- Hamstring curls *(see page 36)*
- The Arrow *(see page 38)*
- Adductors *(see page 39)*
- Hip rolls (1) *(see page 42)*
- Calf strengtheners and raises *(see pages 102–103)*
- Calf stretch *(see pages 128–29)*
- Quads *(see page 101)*
- Upper torso release *(see pages 82–83)*
- Pillow squeeze *(see page 81)*
- Lying pecs *(see page 95)*
- Leg circles *(see pages 104–105)*
- Hamstring and Quad stretches *(see pages 120–23)*
- Tensor fascia lata stretch *(see pages 118–19)*
- Back stretch *(see pages 130–31)*

Quads

If you have ankle weights, you can strap them on for this exercise. Always follow up working on your quads with some Hamstring curls (see page 36).

Contraindications

• If you have knee problems, you may need to reduce the range of movement in this exercise. It's essential that you are able to sit up straight or you will use the wrong leg muscles.

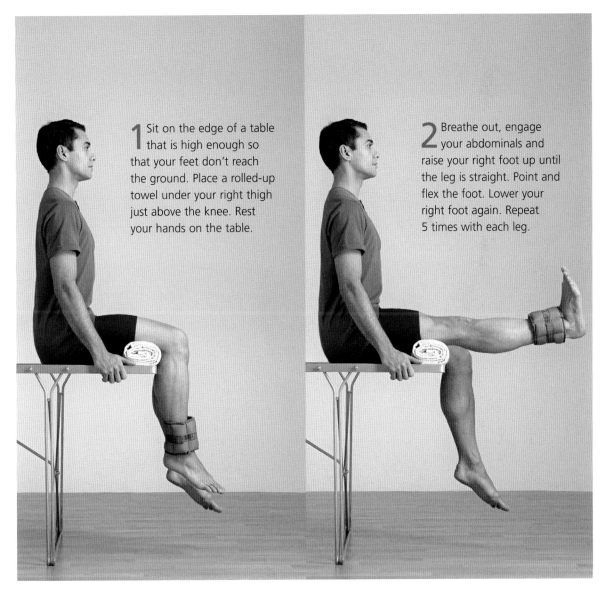

1 Sit on the edge of a table that is high enough so that your feet don't reach the ground. Place a rolled-up towel under your right thigh just above the knee. Rest your hands on the table.

2 Breathe out, engage your abdominals and raise your right foot up until the leg is straight. Point and flex the foot. Lower your right foot again. Repeat 5 times with each leg.

Calf strengtheners

Do this exercise before your run and then follow your run with a calf stretch (see pages 128–29). To work the hamstrings and knees correctly when running, your calves need to be strong and working in conjunction with the movement of the leg.

Contraindications

• As this exercise is done in a non-weight-bearing position, there are no real contraindications.

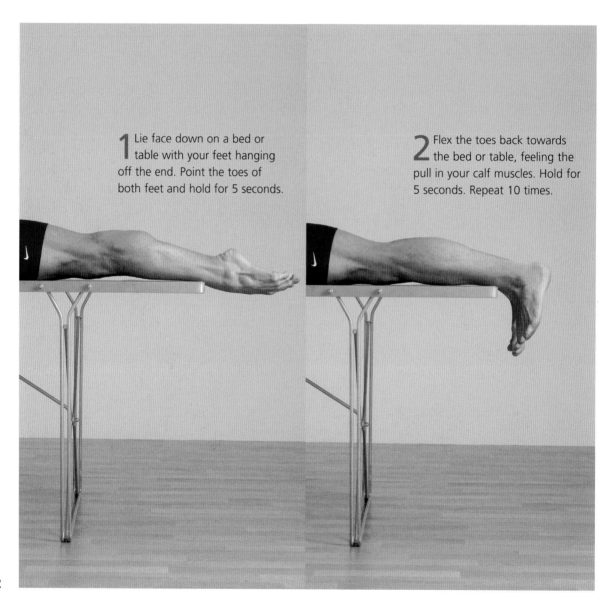

1 Lie face down on a bed or table with your feet hanging off the end. Point the toes of both feet and hold for 5 seconds.

2 Flex the toes back towards the bed or table, feeling the pull in your calf muscles. Hold for 5 seconds. Repeat 10 times.

Calf raises

Keep this movement slow and controlled. For maximum effect, try this standing on a small block or the bottom step of your stairs, where your heels can lower over the edge. This is a great exercise to do before a run.

Contraindications
• Only try this if your ankles are strong enough to hold your body in its correct alignment.

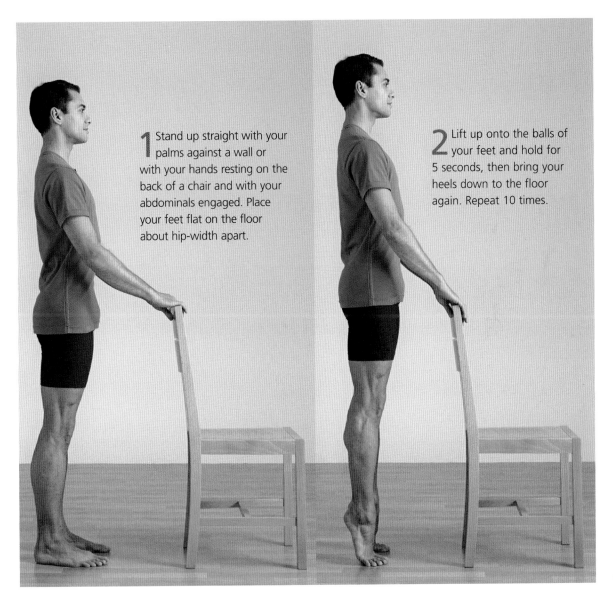

1 Stand up straight with your palms against a wall or with your hands resting on the back of a chair and with your abdominals engaged. Place your feet flat on the floor about hip-width apart.

2 Lift up onto the balls of your feet and hold for 5 seconds, then bring your heels down to the floor again. Repeat 10 times.

Leg circles

This is great for hip mobility, as well as strengthening the abs, glutes and adductors. Start small and slowly increase the size of the circles as you become stronger.

Contraindications

• Note that if you have had a hip replacement, you should avoid crossing your leg across the body. Only try this after asking the advice of your doctor or specialist.

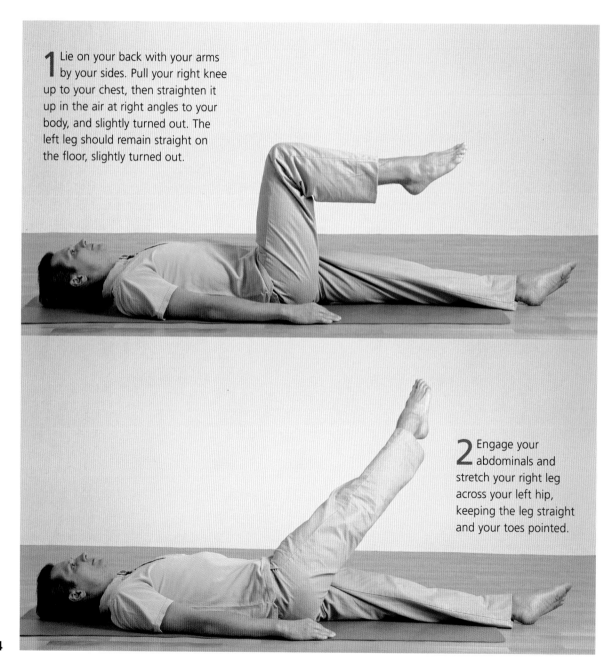

1 Lie on your back with your arms by your sides. Pull your right knee up to your chest, then straighten it up in the air at right angles to your body, and slightly turned out. The left leg should remain straight on the floor, slightly turned out.

2 Engage your abdominals and stretch your right leg across your left hip, keeping the leg straight and your toes pointed.

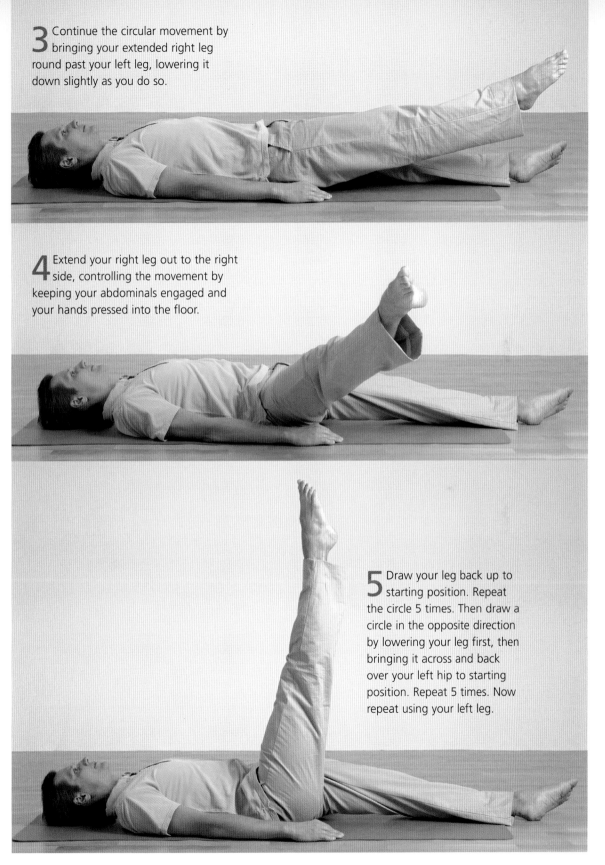

3 Continue the circular movement by bringing your extended right leg round past your left leg, lowering it down slightly as you do so.

4 Extend your right leg out to the right side, controlling the movement by keeping your abdominals engaged and your hands pressed into the floor.

5 Draw your leg back up to starting position. Repeat the circle 5 times. Then draw a circle in the opposite direction by lowering your leg first, then bringing it across and back over your left hip to starting position. Repeat 5 times. Now repeat using your left leg.

Skiing

Very few people ski all year round so it's important to get back in condition – in particular, strengthening the leg muscles – again each winter before you hit the slopes. Retest your equipment every season to check it's in good condition and still fits you well. Are your ski poles the right height so you're not hunched over? And are you using the correct length of skis for your height? Do your skis need a polish? Ski shops and hire centres will be able to advise you on this.

The most common skiing injuries occur as a result of falls. The stronger your core stability and leg muscles, the better your balance and co-ordination should be. There are some Pilates exercises that test balance, such as the Balance test on page 9, and some studios have a narrow beam you can practise walking along by putting one foot in front of the other (it's trickier than it looks). When you do fall, make sure you let go of your ski poles straight away and that the bindings on your skis release easily. Learn how to roll to transmit the shock, and never stretch out a hand to take your weight or try to prevent your fall.

Knee ligaments can take a lot of wear and tear from the twisting and swerving movements of skiing, and injuries can be immediate and acute, or cumulative. Remember: strong quads, hamstrings, calves, hips and back are all that stand between you and knee cartilage surgery.

The workout

- **Static abs** *(see page 31)*
- **Bridging** *(see page 32)*
- **Glute squeezes** *(see page 35)*
- **Hamstring curls** *(see page 36)*
- **The Arrow** *(see page 38)*
- **Adductors** *(see page 39)*
- **Hip rolls (1)** *(see page 42)*
- **Quads** *(see page 101)*
- **Leg circles** *(see pages 104–105)*
- **Swimming** *(see page 55)*
- **The Cat** *(see page 109)*
- **The Dog** *(see pages 110–111)*
- **Wall squats** *(see page 107)*
- **Ankle strengthener** *(see page 107)*
- **Calf stretch** *(see page 128–29)*
- **Balance test** *(see page 9)*

Wall squats

Ankle strengthener

These work a whole range of core stability, hip and leg muscles, and imitate a set of exercises followed in a Pilates studio.

You'll need a rubber exercise band for this – they're available in all major sports shops. I recommend medium strength.

Contraindications
• Reduce the range of movement if you have weak knees.

Contraindications
• If your ankles are weak, use a light-strength band at first.

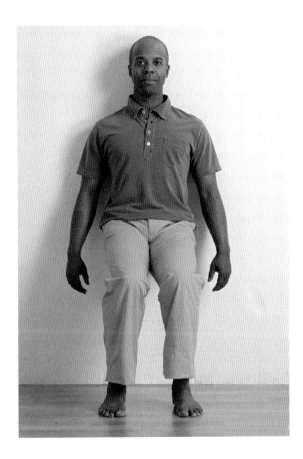

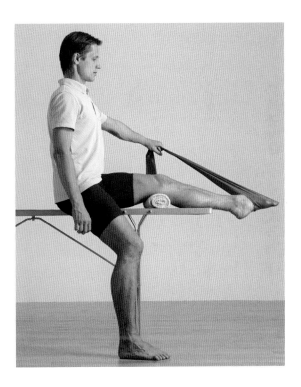

Stand against a wall with your heels a foot-length from the wall. Your feet should be parallel and hip-width apart. Breathe in, engage your abdominals and slide slowly down the wall, letting your knees bend directly over your feet and keeping your heels on the floor. Aim for a right angle at the knees and pause for 10 seconds. Breathe out and slide back up the wall. Repeat 10 times.

Sit on a table with your left foot extended over the edge and a folded towel placed under your knee. Rest your right foot on the floor. Place your flexi-band round your left foot, covering your toes. Hold onto the ends of the flexi-band and pull it taut. Point and flex your foot against the resistance of the flexi-band, keeping your toes straight so the ankle is doing the work. Next, take the flexi-band in your left hand and pull it roughly 45 degrees out from the centre line to your left side. Point and flex your foot keeping your leg still so that the only movement is in the ankle joint. Repeat the sequence 5 times on each leg.

Swimming

Swimming is one of the safest of sports because your joints are not carrying your body weight or absorbing impact from your feet jarring against the ground. However, swimming with incorrect techniques can, over time, lead to joint pain or wear and tear. If you haven't taken swimming lessons since school, it can be worth booking a session with a professional who can assess and correct your strokes.

In freestyle and breaststroke, a common error can be holding your head either too high or too low in the water; too high will cause you to arch your lower back and compress the vertebrae of your lumbar spine, while too low can strain your arms and shoulders. In freestyle, breathe on both sides and try to limit the side-to-side rolling of your body as much as possible. In breaststroke, knee injuries can occur as a result of poor kicking technique, which puts strain on the kneecap. With all these problems the pain will probably develop gradually, over time, rather than become acute after one swim.

The other vulnerable joint when swimming is the shoulder, which has to achieve a different range of movement for each stroke. It's important to keep the supportive muscles round the rotator cuff strong and, as with other sports, warm up before you start. Watch that you don't develop tendencies towards kyphosis, with rounded shoulders and shortened chest muscles. Whichever stroke you have been using in a session, stretch in the opposite direction when you are cooling down.

The workout

- Static abs *(see page 31)*
- Bridging *(see page 32)*
- Glute squeezes *(see page 35)*
- Hamstring curls *(see page 36)*
- The Arrow *(see page 38)*
- Adductors *(see page 39)*
- Hip rolls (1) *(see page 42)*
- Double leg stretch *(see pages 62–63)*
- Leg circles *(see pages 104–105)*
- Chest opening exercise *(see page 90)*
- Chest opening exercise with circle *(see page 91)*
- Twisting with a pole *(see page 85)*
- Swimming *(see page 55)*
- The Dog *(see pages 110–111)*
- The Cat *(see page 109)*

The Cat

This is a good strengthening exercise for the lumbar spine and abdominal muscles. Make sure you get a full spinal stretch from the tailbone all the way up to the neck, using a smooth rippling movement.

Contraindications

- Be careful during this exercise if you have knee, shoulder or wrist problems.
- Keep the curve to a minimum in step 3 if you have lumbar weakness.

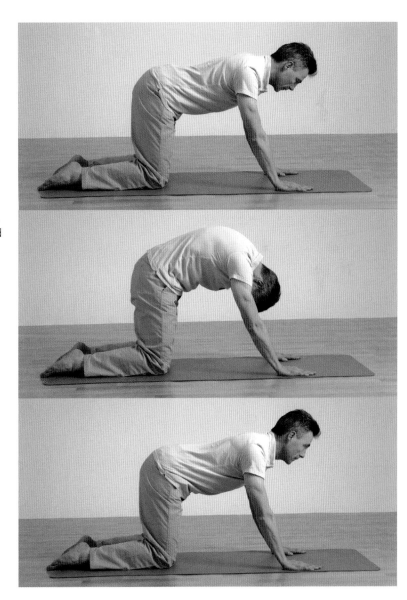

1 Kneel on all fours with your hands shoulder-width apart and your knees about hip-width apart, as for the Dog. Hold your head so that your spine is in its natural curves.

2 Breathe in and round your back upwards while letting your head drop down and feeling the stretch right through your spine.

3 Breathe out, engage your abdominals, then scoop your back down into a curve and raise your head up. Repeat steps 2 and 3 in a smooth, flowing movement 10 times.

The Dog

The aim is to keep your back utterly straight while you move your limbs in this exercise. In the Pilates studio, we sometimes balance a pole on the back where it will fall off if the torso is not kept stable.

Contraindications

- Take care if you have weakness in the knees, shoulders or wrists.
- Those with weak wrists may find it helps to roll up a small towel and rest their hands on this instead of flat on the floor.
- In step 4, place a cushion between your calves and the backs of your legs if it feels tight.

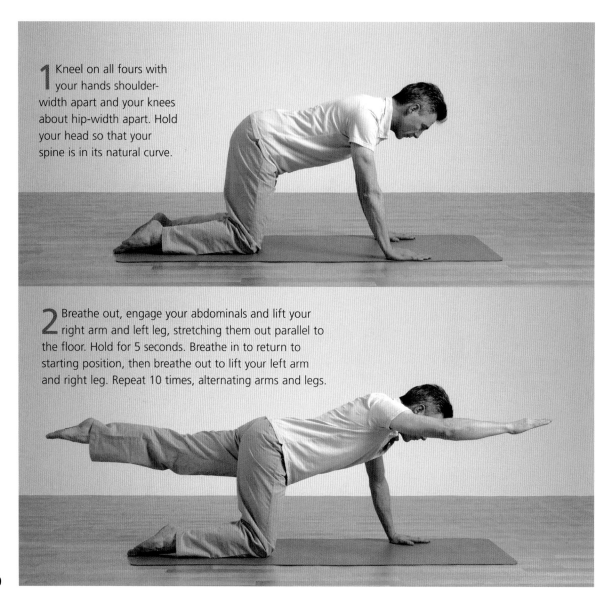

1 Kneel on all fours with your hands shoulder-width apart and your knees about hip-width apart. Hold your head so that your spine is in its natural curve.

2 Breathe out, engage your abdominals and lift your right arm and left leg, stretching them out parallel to the floor. Hold for 5 seconds. Breathe in to return to starting position, then breathe out to lift your left arm and right leg. Repeat 10 times, alternating arms and legs.

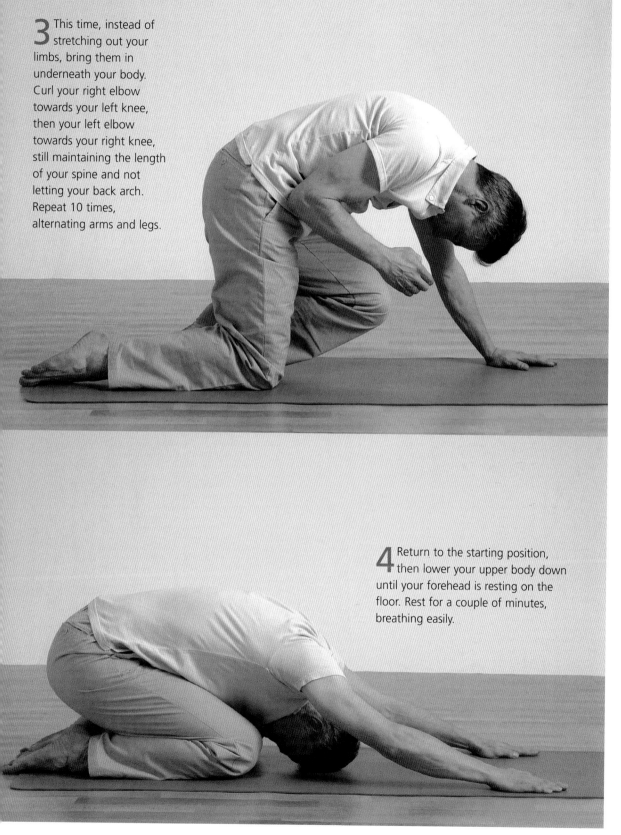

3 This time, instead of stretching out your limbs, bring them in underneath your body. Curl your right elbow towards your left knee, then your left elbow towards your right knee, still maintaining the length of your spine and not letting your back arch. Repeat 10 times, alternating arms and legs.

4 Return to the starting position, then lower your upper body down until your forehead is resting on the floor. Rest for a couple of minutes, breathing easily.

Tennis and squash

Make no mistake: while tennis and squash are a great aerobic workout and a good muscle strengthener, they require a high degree of general fitness and a good balance of strength in opposing muscle groups. It's definitely worth getting a professional coach to check your serve, backhand and forehand, as incorrect movements can cause some nasty injuries, both acute and chronic. Use your Pilates session after playing a game to stretch out the racquet side and strengthen the other side to try and combat any potential one-sidedness that could develop.

The correct equipment is vital. Choose a large-headed tennis racquet so there will be fewer off-centre hits that create vibration up the arm. The strings shouldn't be too tight, as this will also affect vibration. There's a formula for getting the correct racquet grip size. Find the midpoint of your palm, where a line drawn from the centre of your middle finger would intersect with one drawn across from the top of the point where your thumb meets your palm. Measure from that central point to the end of your ring finger and that's the circumference of racquet grip you need.

Your shoes should be a good fit, with proper arch support and enough flexibility for backwards, forwards and sideways movements. Be aware that hard courts cause more impact on the joints and you need more shoulder strength because the ball moves faster.

Perhaps the most important advice is only to play against people who are more or less at the same level as you. Don't take on the county champion if you're just used to friendly knockabouts on a Saturday morning, or you could find yourself overstretched – literally!

The workout

- **Static abs** *(see page 31)*
- **Bridging** *(see page 32)*
- **Glute squeezes** *(see page 35)*
- **Hamstring curls** *(see page 36)*
- **The Arrow** *(see page 38)*
- **Adductors** *(see page 39)*
- **Hip rolls (1)** *(see page 42)*
- **Push-ups** *(see pages 72–73)*
- **The Saw** *(see page 64)*
- **Rowing (2)** *(see pages 68–69)*
- **Single leg teaser** *(see pages 66–67)*
- **Arm weights** *(see page 78)*
- **Lying pecs** *(see page 95)*
- **Arm and elbow circles** *(see pages 76–77)*
- **Chest opening exercise** *(see page 90)*
- **Chest opening with circle exercise** *(see page 91)*
- **Shoulder stretch** *(see page 113)*
- **The Windmill** *(see pages 114–15)*
- **Wrist strengthener** *(see page 95)*

Shoulder stretch

The beauty of this stretch is that you can do it wherever there is a doorway or where two walls meet at a corner. It's good to do after a match to counteract all that forward shoulder movement.

Contraindications

• If you have upper spine problems or shoulder impingement, you may need to reduce the range of movement in this exercise.

1 Stand in front of the doorway with your right arm extended at shoulder height with your palm pressing into the wall. Engage your abdominals, then walk your feet around and away from your arm, so that your shoulder is stretched backwards. Hold for 5 seconds then walk back again. Repeat 5 times with each shoulder.

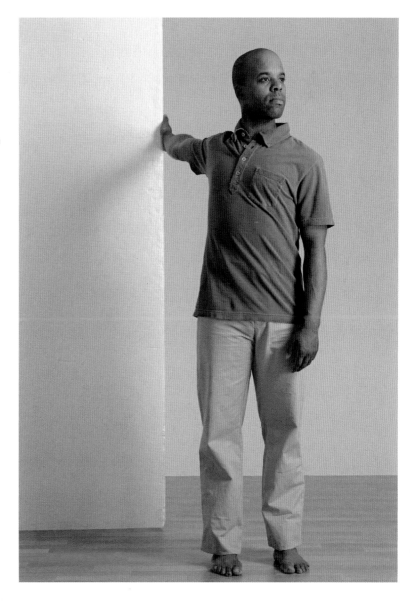

The Windmill

Do this exercise very slowly and smoothly, using the recommended breathing pattern for maximum results. Keep your arms straight throughout and only move within your comfort zone.

Contraindications

* Don't do this exercise if you have shoulder mobility impingement.
* If you have neck or upper spine weakness, don't put the towel under your back – but do use it if you are just stiff in the shoulderblade region.

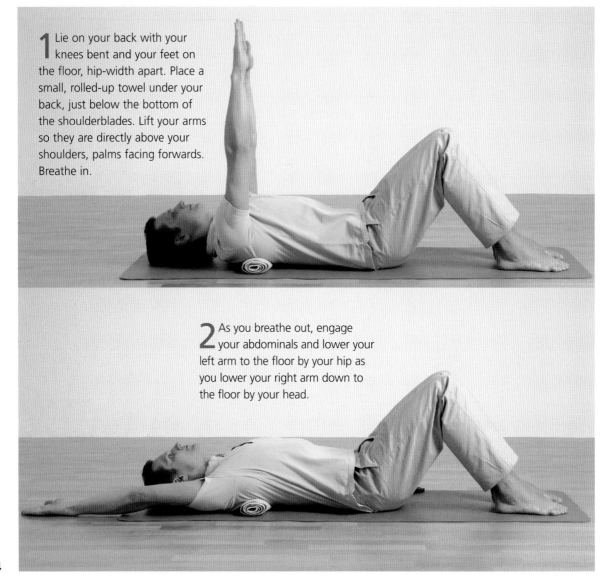

1 Lie on your back with your knees bent and your feet on the floor, hip-width apart. Place a small, rolled-up towel under your back, just below the bottom of the shoulderblades. Lift your arms so they are directly above your shoulders, palms facing forwards. Breathe in.

2 As you breathe out, engage your abdominals and lower your left arm to the floor by your hip as you lower your right arm down to the floor by your head.

3 Breathe in as you bring both arms back up to the centre, then repeat in the opposite direction, bringing your right arm down to rest by your hip and your left arm by your head. Do 10 repetitions each way.

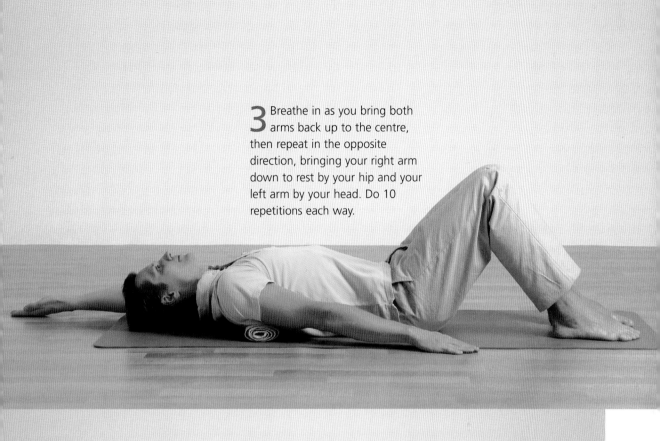

4 Now bring your left arm down by your hip and your right arm by your head and draw a circle round the sides of your body with your hands. Sweep your left arm along the floor up towards, then alongside your head and your right arm along the floor down towards, then alongside your hips. When your arms reach shoulder level, pause to breathe in and turn your left hand palm down and your right hand palm up. Bring them back up to centre. Repeat 10 times in each direction.

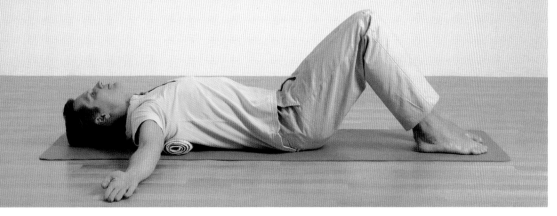

Chapter 6
Stretching

After any exercise, stretching as part of your 'cool down' helps to ease out any muscle tension that may have developed. It's a good idea to do some stretches every day to release tension in the muscles, giving the joints a wider range of movement and thus helping you to become more supple. Flexible, stretched muscles will resist stresses and strains much more easily than stiff, unstretched ones. Surely you can spare five minutes every morning to wake up your muscles? What could be more important?

Adductors stretch

Stretch the inner thigh muscles immediately after stretching your hamstrings and quads.

1 Lie on your back with your tailbone close to a wall and your legs resting against the wall in a wide 'V' shape. Find a position that feels comfortable.

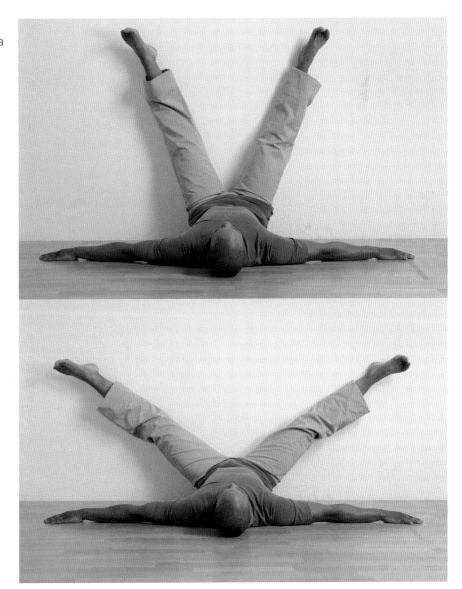

2 Relax and let gravity pull your legs wider, creating a stretch in the inner thighs. Breathing out, soften your knees to slightly bend them, then straighten them again. To get a good stretch lie in this position for at least a minute.

Tensor Fascia Lata stretches

The TFL is a small but important muscle with a long ligament down the outsides of your legs. This particular stretch is especially useful for footballers, whose leg muscles tend to become more developed on one side than the other.

Caution
To help stabilize the table, ask someone to hold down the opposite end.

On a table

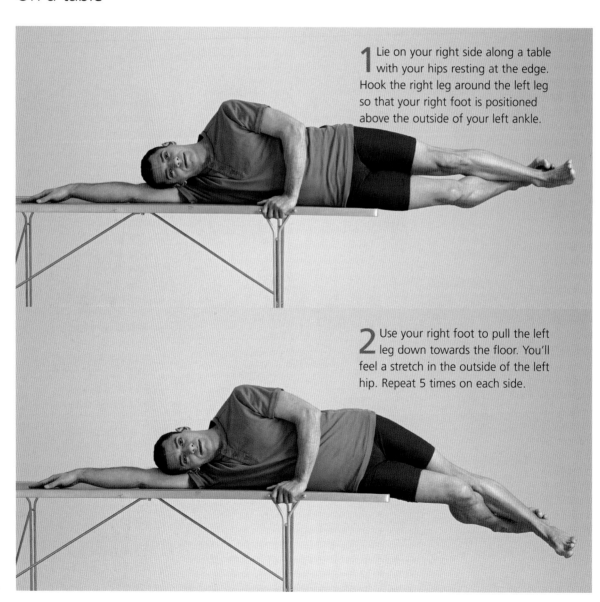

1 Lie on your right side along a table with your hips resting at the edge. Hook the right leg around the left leg so that your right foot is positioned above the outside of your left ankle.

2 Use your right foot to pull the left leg down towards the floor. You'll feel a stretch in the outside of the left hip. Repeat 5 times on each side.

Standing

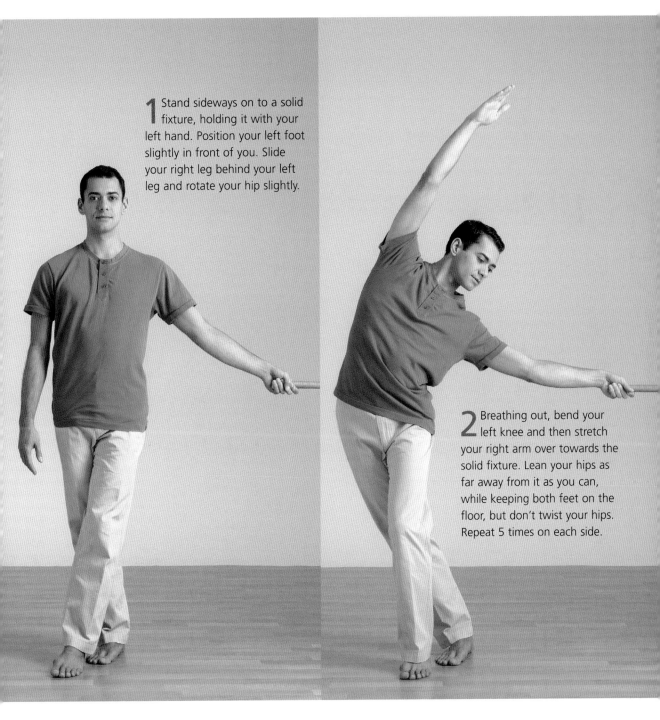

1 Stand sideways on to a solid fixture, holding it with your left hand. Position your left foot slightly in front of you. Slide your right leg behind your left leg and rotate your hip slightly.

2 Breathing out, bend your left knee and then stretch your right arm over towards the solid fixture. Lean your hips as far away from it as you can, while keeping both feet on the floor, but don't twist your hips. Repeat 5 times on each side.

Hamstring stretches

These fibrous muscles down the backs of the legs are particularly prone to tightness and should be stretched after any activities that involve running. Here are two methods I recommend.

Against a wall

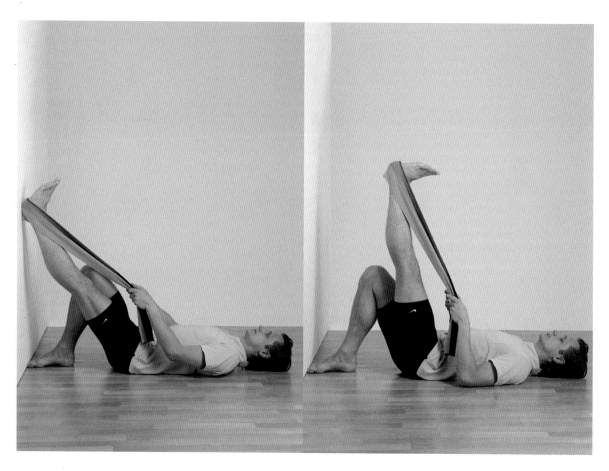

1 Lie on your back near a wall. Loop a flexi-band or towel round your left foot and rest it against the wall so that it is at an angle of roughly 60 degrees to the floor. Bend your right leg. Hold the ends of the flexi-band in each hand. Breathe in and press your heel into the wall. Hold for 4 seconds.

2 Breathing out, use the flexi-band to pull your heel away from the wall. Keep your leg straight, feeling the pull down the back of your thigh. To get even more stretch, point and flex your foot. Repeat 10 times with each leg.

On a table

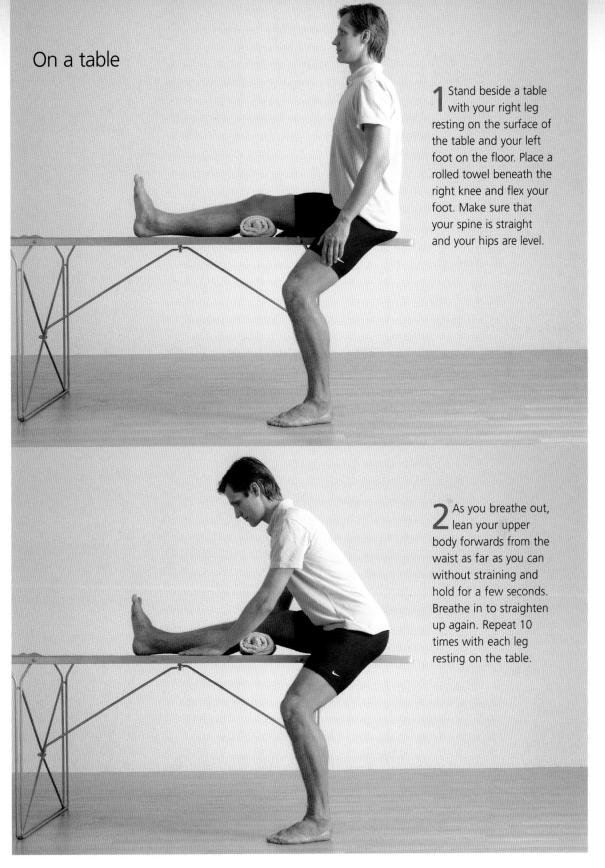

1 Stand beside a table with your right leg resting on the surface of the table and your left foot on the floor. Place a rolled towel beneath the right knee and flex your foot. Make sure that your spine is straight and your hips are level.

2 As you breathe out, lean your upper body forwards from the waist as far as you can without straining and hold for a few seconds. Breathe in to straighten up again. Repeat 10 times with each leg resting on the table.

Quads stretches

These front-of-thigh stretches are particularly useful for cyclists. Once again, I've given you two stretches to choose from – one passive and one active.

On your back

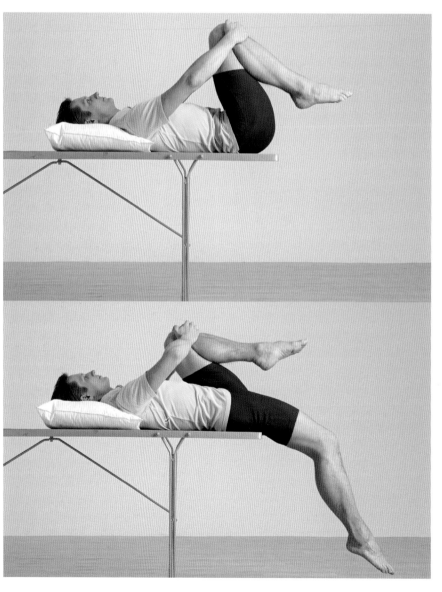

1 Lie down on a table with a cushion supporting your neck, shoulders and head. Draw both knees up to your chest. Adjust your position so that your tailbone is just at the edge of the table.

2 Breathe out and engage your abdominals as you gently lower your right leg towards the floor, making sure that your lower back remains on the table. Hold for a few seconds. Keeping your back pressed into the table, breathe in and lift your right leg back up to your chest. Breathing out, lower your left leg. Repeat 10 times with each leg.

On your front

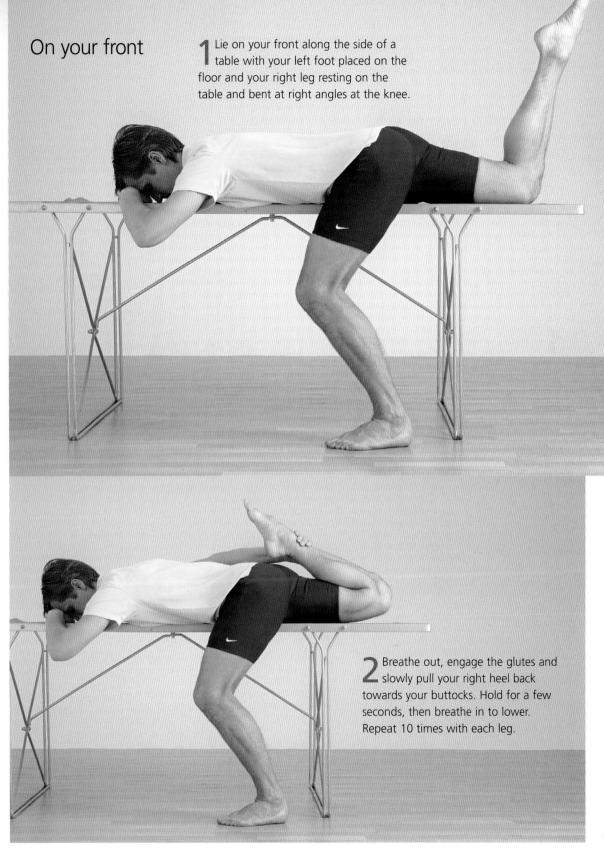

1 Lie on your front along the side of a table with your left foot placed on the floor and your right leg resting on the table and bent at right angles at the knee.

2 Breathe out, engage the glutes and slowly pull your right heel back towards your buttocks. Hold for a few seconds, then breathe in to lower. Repeat 10 times with each leg.

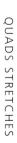

Abdominal stretches

Both of the abdominal stretch exercises I recommend here have been described elsewhere in the book, but when you are using them in a stretching session they can be taken a bit further.

The Cobra (2)

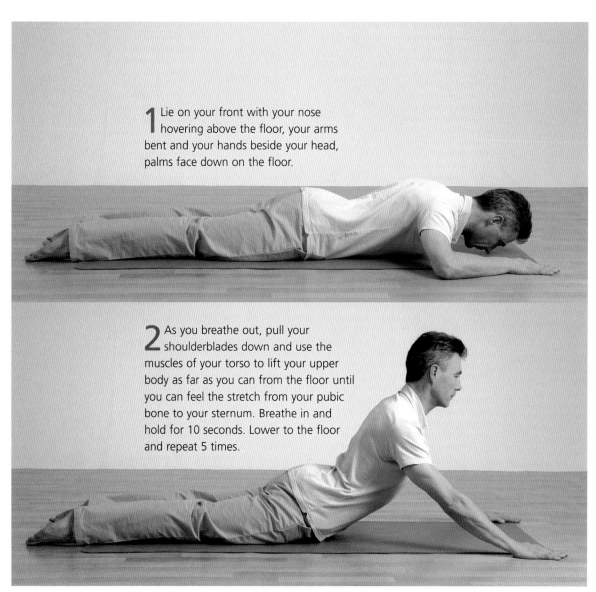

1 Lie on your front with your nose hovering above the floor, your arms bent and your hands beside your head, palms face down on the floor.

2 As you breathe out, pull your shoulderblades down and use the muscles of your torso to lift your upper body as far as you can from the floor until you can feel the stretch from your pubic bone to your sternum. Breathe in and hold for 10 seconds. Lower to the floor and repeat 5 times.

Hip rolls (2)

1 Lie on your back with your knees bent at right angles in the air above your hips. Keep your feet and legs together and extend your arms out by your sides at shoulder level.

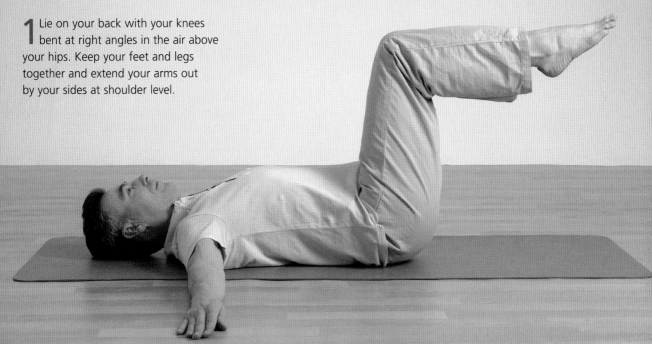

2 As you breathe out, use your abdominals to lower your knees to the left. Let your right hip lift, but keep your shoulders firmly on the floor. Turn your head to the right. Hold the stretch for a few seconds. Breathe in to come up to centre, then breathe out to lower your knees to the right, turning your head to the left. Repeat 5 times in each direction.

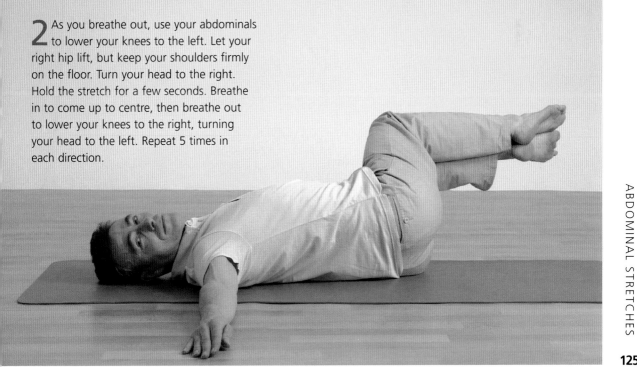

Quadratus Lumborum stretches

The QL muscles are down the sides of your torso. In Pilates, we don't usually do side stretches without using some kind of anchor to prevent you overstretching your muscles.

Sitting down

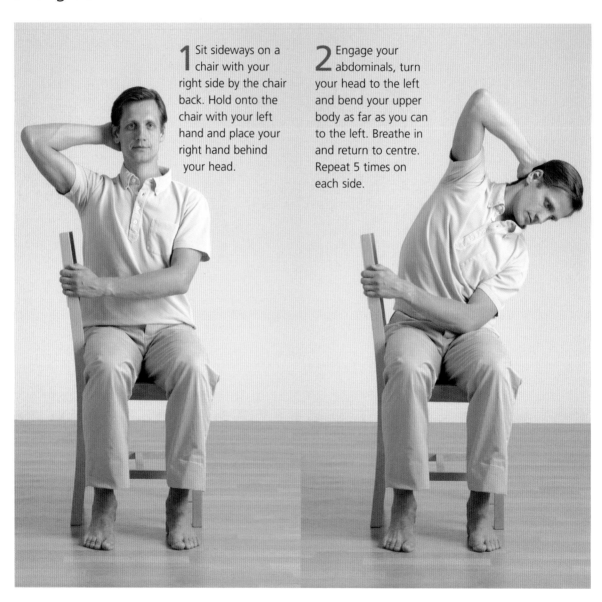

1 Sit sideways on a chair with your right side by the chair back. Hold onto the chair with your left hand and place your right hand behind your head.

2 Engage your abdominals, turn your head to the left and bend your upper body as far as you can to the left. Breathe in and return to centre. Repeat 5 times on each side.

Standing

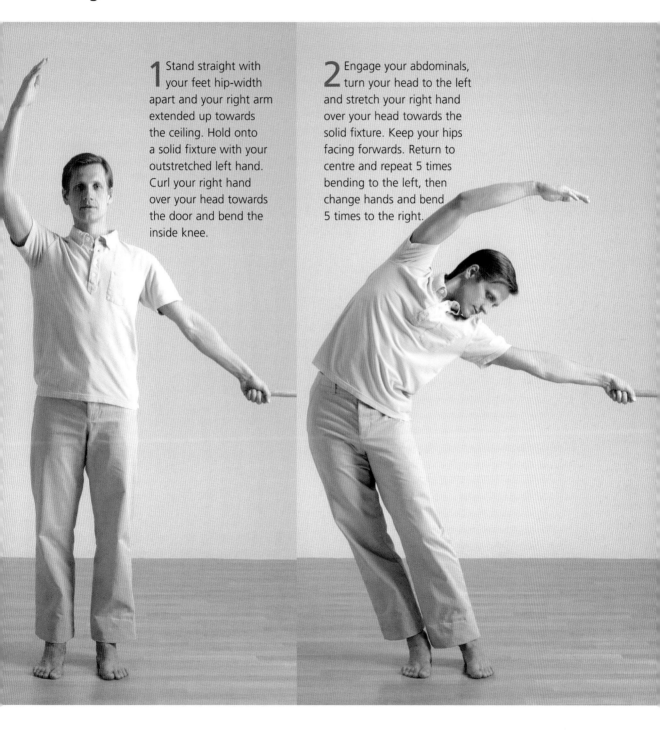

1 Stand straight with your feet hip-width apart and your right arm extended up towards the ceiling. Hold onto a solid fixture with your outstretched left hand. Curl your right hand over your head towards the door and bend the inside knee.

2 Engage your abdominals, turn your head to the left and stretch your right hand over your head towards the solid fixture. Keep your hips facing forwards. Return to centre and repeat 5 times bending to the left, then change hands and bend 5 times to the right.

Calf stretches

Running, skiing and cycling all put a lot of strain on the calf muscles, therefore they should be stretched before and after these activities or any sport that involves running.

With a chair

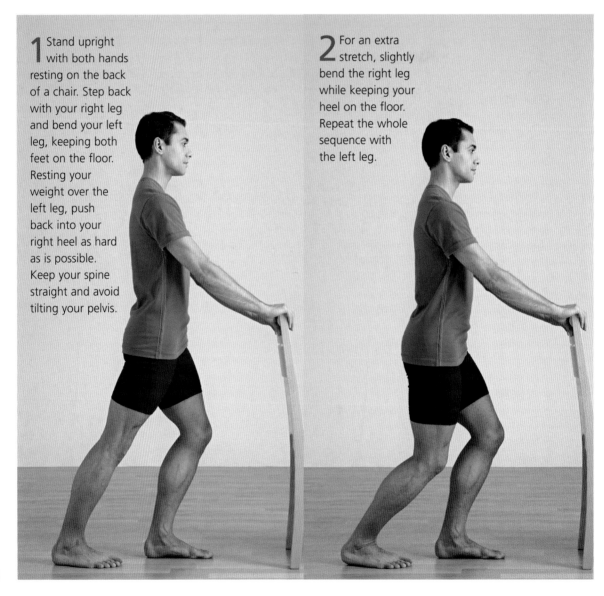

1 Stand upright with both hands resting on the back of a chair. Step back with your right leg and bend your left leg, keeping both feet on the floor. Resting your weight over the left leg, push back into your right heel as hard as is possible. Keep your spine straight and avoid tilting your pelvis.

2 For an extra stretch, slightly bend the right leg while keeping your heel on the floor. Repeat the whole sequence with the left leg.

Against a chair leg

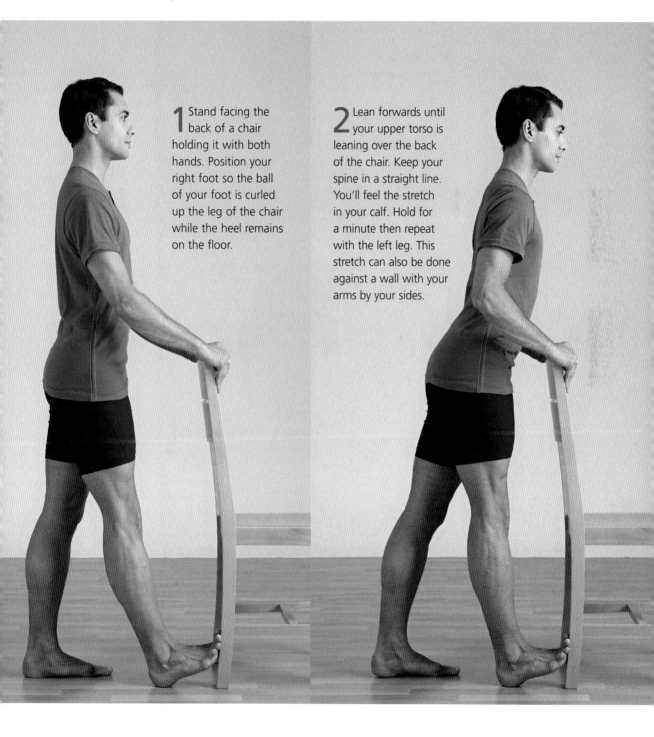

1 Stand facing the back of a chair holding it with both hands. Position your right foot so the ball of your foot is curled up the leg of the chair while the heel remains on the floor.

2 Lean forwards until your upper torso is leaning over the back of the chair. Keep your spine in a straight line. You'll feel the stretch in your calf. Hold for a minute then repeat with the left leg. This stretch can also be done against a wall with your arms by your sides.

Back stretch

There are some back stretching exercises earlier in the book (see Back stretch on pages 40–41, Spine stretch on page 57 and Rolling like a ball on page 53). Use one of them, or try this Spine rolldown as part of your stretching session.

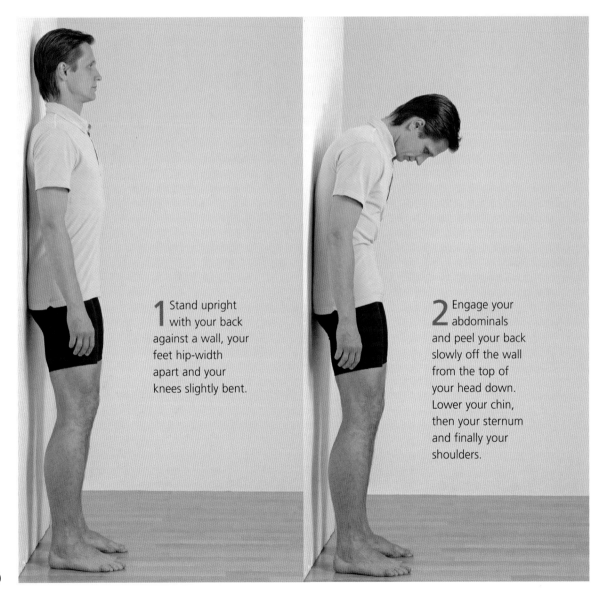

1 Stand upright with your back against a wall, your feet hip-width apart and your knees slightly bent.

2 Engage your abdominals and peel your back slowly off the wall from the top of your head down. Lower your chin, then your sternum and finally your shoulders.

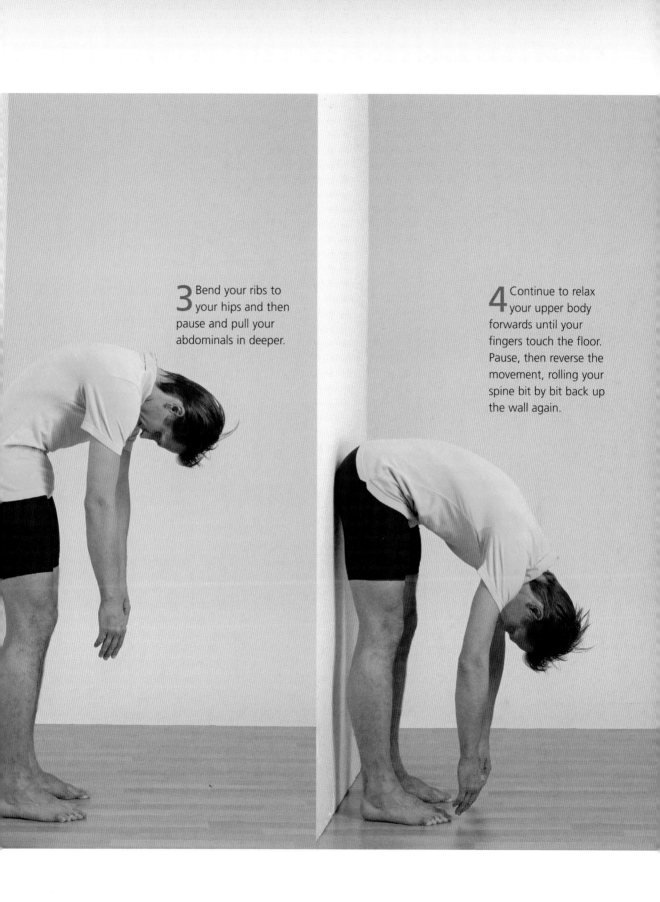

3 Bend your ribs to your hips and then pause and pull your abdominals in deeper.

4 Continue to relax your upper body forwards until your fingers touch the floor. Pause, then reverse the movement, rolling your spine bit by bit back up the wall again.

Shoulder stretches

You can do these simple exercises while sitting at your desk at work as well as in your sports warm-ups and cool-downs while standing. To get the maximum benefit, maintain good posture throughout.

Pulling the elbow

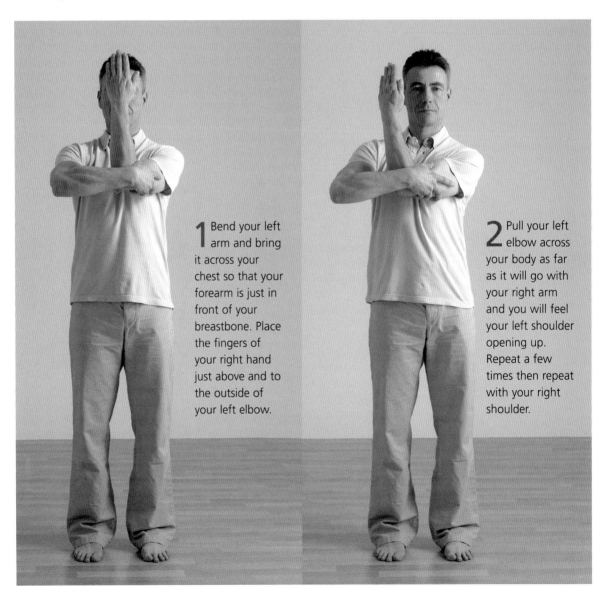

1 Bend your left arm and bring it across your chest so that your forearm is just in front of your breastbone. Place the fingers of your right hand just above and to the outside of your left elbow.

2 Pull your left elbow across your body as far as it will go with your right arm and you will feel your left shoulder opening up. Repeat a few times then repeat with your right shoulder.

Hands behind your back

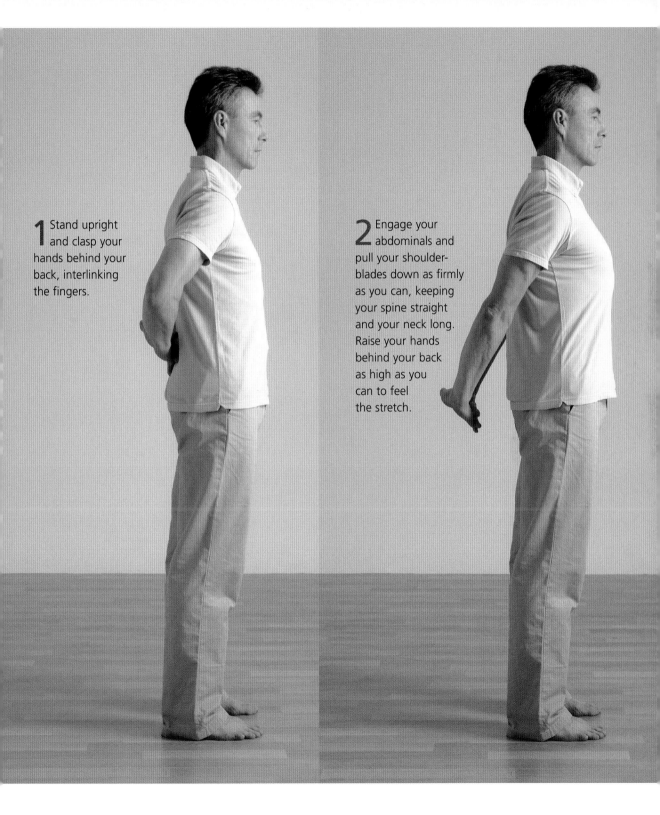

1 Stand upright and clasp your hands behind your back, interlinking the fingers.

2 Engage your abdominals and pull your shoulder-blades down as firmly as you can, keeping your spine straight and your neck long. Raise your hands behind your back as high as you can to feel the stretch.

Neck stretch

Be gentle with these stretches if your neck muscles are feeling tight. Rather than pulling your head down, think of letting gravity do the stretching. Keep your spinal alignment – don't move your upper body into the stretch.

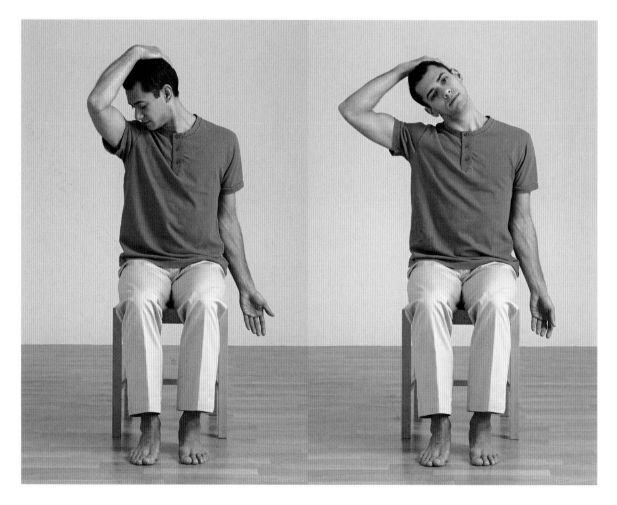

1 Sit up straight on a chair with your feet flat on the floor. Place your right hand over the top of your head and turn your head to face into your right upper arm. Hold your left arm straight down by your side with the palm rotated outwards so it faces forwards.

2 Lean the weight of your head over, pulling on it very gently with your right hand. Rotate your left hand so the palm is facing forwards, stretch your arm towards the floor, and you'll feel the stretch in the left side of your neck.

3 Repeat the stretch with your left hand over your head and your right arm stretching towards the floor.

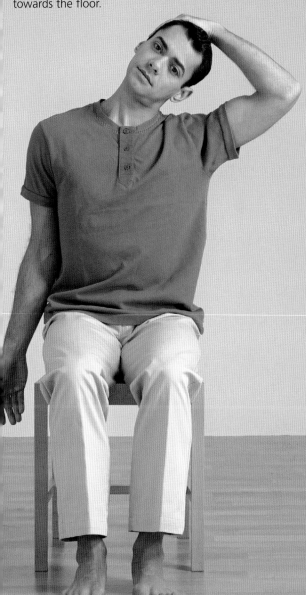

4 Place both hands at the back of your skull and pull your head forwards, at the same time resisting the pull so that you feel the stretch in the muscles at the back of your neck.

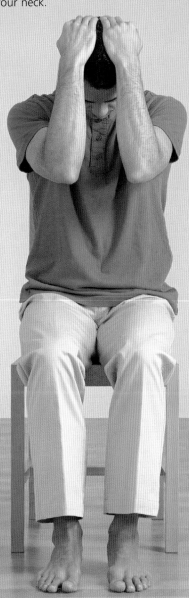

Your lifestyle

One of the reasons for the popularity of Pilates is its flexibility. The stretches in this chapter can be used whenever you need them: after sport, after a tough day at work, or first thing in the morning to loosen up your joints for the day ahead. Similarly, Pilates workouts don't need to be full, structured routines every time. Here are some ways of making Pilates part of an all-round healthy lifestyle.

Keep moving

I generally advise clients to get an hour-long exercise workout every second day, either Pilates or some kind of aerobic exercise or sport. If you can't find time for long sessions, do a 15- to 20-minute session every day instead. Make sure that you cover a range of exercises for different parts of the body instead of focusing on a few favourites each time. In my experience, the ones you don't like doing are probably the ones you need the most.

The rest of the time, keep as active as you can: walk upstairs rather than taking the lift or the elevator, go and talk to colleagues on another floor instead of e-mailing them, borrow someone's dog to walk, or use your lunch hour to march round the park. We're not designed to be sedentary creatures and our bodies slump, muscles shorten and joints degenerate if they're not used regularly.

Work out how to incorporate Pilates into your routine. It doesn't require time-consuming trips to the gym but can be done at home in the evening, at work during your lunch hour (so long as you have a relatively private office), or in hotel rooms when you're travelling. The gentle pace of the exercises is very calming, but at the same time they provide the feel-good endorphin release that makes exercise so rewarding.

During the day, get into the habit of engaging your abdominals and glutes while you're walking to get instantly better posture. Pull your navel to your spine and engage your pelvic floor while watching TV. Keep correcting your posture according to the principles I explained in chapter 1 and I guarantee you will feel better and look better very quickly.

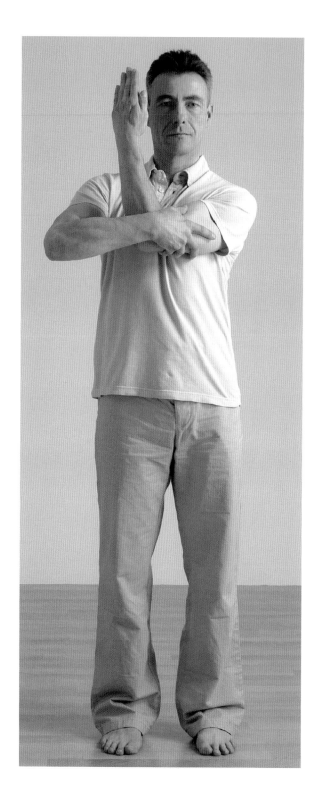

Stress-busting

If you frequently find yourself rushing to complete umpteen tasks in record time, stop and consider whether it's really necessary. What will happen if you miss that deadline? Unless you're a fireman, an ambulance driver or an A & E doctor, no one is likely to die if you're late. 'My boss would kill me,' some say – but of course he wouldn't. You could be killing yourself, though, because chronic stress takes a huge toll on the body over time.

When we're stressed, adrenaline is released, the heart beats faster, blood is diverted to the limbs in case we need to run from danger, kidney function slows down, the pupils dilate, lungs take in extra oxygen, the liver releases more fat and sugar for energy, digestion slows or stops, the mouth feels dry and sweating increases. This would be fine, and all very useful, if we had to run away from a sabre-toothed tiger, but maintaining your body on 'high alert' day in and day out depletes your resources of nutrients and hormones leading to a state known as adrenal exhaustion – basically running on empty. In this state, our stress tolerance decreases and we are much less effective at decision-making, creativity and logic than our non-stressed equivalent.

What could you do to decrease your stress levels and improve your work–life balance? The answer will be individual but you may find that some slight adjustments would help. We all need to find our own way of clicking a switch after work so that we don't take problems home with us, and many men find that exercise is the key. My Pilates studio often fills up with wrung-out, grey-faced business types at the close of office hours, and they leave in a much more mellow frame of mind. The exercises seem to provide the perfect antidote to the frenzied 21st century lifestyle.

Eat well

What you eat and drink is obviously an important part of maintaining a healthy lifestyle. There are far too many diet programmes out there already, so I'm not going to add my tuppence-worth except to remind you that your joints really suffer when you're overweight. The media is full of talking heads telling us that we should be eating those five portions of fruit and veg a day and opting for fresh, unprocessed foods with a high fibre content, but when you're stressed, the best intentions can quickly go out the window. Surveys show that stress makes us crave high-sugar, high-fat, calorie-laden junk foods that give a quick energy burst and leave us depleted soon afterwards – and craving that next chocolate bar. To break the cycle, opt for low-GI, slow-burn wholefoods that will provide a steady energy release for a few hours after eating.

Unless you've had your head in the sand, you should be aware that the government recommended alcohol intake is no more than 3 units a day for men (where a unit is a 125ml glass of wine, a half pint of beer or a single measure of spirits). There are many health reasons why you shouldn't exceed this, but vanity may provide a greater incentive. Alcohol calories are quickly converted to sugar in the digestive system and they go straight to the waistline without providing any nutritional benefits. My tip is to remind yourself of this fact by always pulling your stomach in before reaching for that glass. I do it myself and it works!

Sleep well

Finally, your general health is hugely influenced by the quality of your sleep, so we all need to find ways to get restful nights. Here are my thoughts on the subject.
• Buy a good medium-to-firm support mattress, and change it at least every ten years.
• Choose a pillow that's the correct height to keep your neck in line with your spine.
• If you suffer from lower back pain, sleep on your side and slip a pillow between your legs to maintain pelvic alignment so there's no pulling on the lumbar spine.
• Make sure you have been physically active during the day, so that your muscles are tired.

Glossary

Abdominals – three muscle groups in the abdomen that extend from the rib cage to the pelvis: the rectus abdominus, the transverse abdominals and the obliques. Pilates abdominal exercises target all three.

Abduction – a movement away from the centre line of the body. The muscles in the arms and legs used for this action are known as abductors.

Adduction – a movement towards the centre line of the body. The muscles in the arms and legs used for this action are known as adductors.

Aerobic exercise – exercise that raises the heart beat and makes you breathe harder to get more oxygen to the muscles. Running, cycling and swimming are all aerobic if you work hard enough.

Cervical spine – the part of the spine in the neck area.

Core stability – muscle strength round the middle of the body that helps to hold the pelvis and spine in correct alignment and protect the body from injury. Core stability is one of the key goals in Pilates.

Deltoids – muscles across the shoulders that move the arms up and down and to the sides.

Engaging the abdominals – pulling your stomach muscles towards your spine. This instruction is often given at the beginning of a Pilates exercise.

Extension – extending. If you are asked to extend an arm or a leg in an exercise, it means that you should straighten it.

Flexion – bending. If you are asked to flex your foot in an exercise, you should bend it back towards your shin.

Glutes – the large gluteus maximus muscles across the bottom help to straighten the hip and rotate the hip joint outwards. They are also used to help raise the torso up from moves such as a forward bend and move the legs backwards.

Hamstrings – muscles down the backs of the thighs that help to bend the knee and straighten the hip. It's important to keep these muscles strong if you want to avoid the risk of knee injuries.

Intercostal muscles – muscles between the ribs, used for inhalation and forced exhalation.

Isometric – a movement that contracts the muscle without shortening it.

Kyphosis – pronounced forwards curve of the upper back, creating a humped appearance. Pilates can help to relieve the pain associated with kyphosis by strengthening the upper and middle back muscles.

Latissimus dorsi (lats) – muscles of the mid back that hold the shoulderblades down, pull the arms backwards and rotate them inwards.

Lordosis – pronounced curvature of the lower back that causes the stomach and bottom to stick out. Pilates can help to relieve the problems associated with lordosis by strengthening the stomach, glute, hamstring and pelvic floor muscles.

Lumbar spine – the part of the spine found in the lower back.

Multifidis – the deep muscles in the lower abdomen.

Muscular strength – the ability of a muscle to exert maximum force to overcome a resistance.

Obliques – muscles round the sides of the waist that help to turn the body to the sides.

Pectorals – the muscles of the chest area that are used in moving the arms forwards and pushing away from the body.

Pelvic alignment – the pelvis can be tilted backwards and forwards, but for daily movements and activities it should be held by the surrounding muscles in an alignment that doesn't put any strain on the spine. Poor posture and sitting cross-legged affects pelvic alignment.

Pelvic floor – the hammock of muscles between the legs that supports the bladder and bowels. It is important to keep these muscles strong in order to promote core stability.

Quadratus lumborum – stabilizing muscles located on either side of the back at waist level, orginating from the inferior border of the 12th rib.

Quadriceps (quads) – muscles at the fronts of the thighs that straighten the knee. These are used for activities such as walking, running, cycling, day-to-day activities such as standing up from a chair, and in many exercises.

Range of movement – the amount that a joint can rotate comfortably without strain.

Rectus abdominus – a muscle running from the breastbone down to the pubic bone that is used when bending the body forwards.

Scoliosis – sideways curvature of the spine, often in an 'S' shape. Pilates can help to strengthen the weaker side of the body and create strong abdominal and pelvic muscles to help the spine to straighten.

Serratus anterior – muscles in the sides of the body that pull the shoulderblades forward.

Sternum – breastbone.

Thoracic spine – the part of the spine in the mid back.

Transverse abdominals – these hold your internal organs in place and are used in Pilates to pull your stomach towards your back.

Trapezius – a diamond-shaped muscle across the upper back for raising the shoulders, rotating the shoulder-blades and lifting your arms above your head.

Index

Acknowledgements

Alan Herdman would like to thank the models for their dedication and hard work: Denzil Bailey, Gilles Crawford, Thomas Edur and Joshua Tuifua. He would also like to thank Richard Burnes for grooming.

Executive Editor Jo Godfreywood
Editor Camilla Davis
Executive Art Editor Leigh Jones
Designer Martin Topping
Photographer Paul Forrester
Production Manager Louise Hall